TWO GIRLFRIENDS GET REAL ABOUT COSMETIC SURGERY

D1401598

TWO GIRLFRIENDS GET REAL ABOUT COSMETIC SURGERY

CHARLEE GANNY
AND SUSAN J. COLLINI

To you
Charlee Ganny
Susan J. Collini

BOOKS

RENAISSANCE BOOKS
Los Angeles

Library of Congress Cataloging-in-Publication Data

Collini, Susan J.
    Two girlfriends get real about cosmetic surgery / Susan J. Collini and Charlee Ganny.
        p. cm.
    Includes bibliographical references and index.
    ISBN 1-58063-127-4 (trade paper)
        1. Surgery, Plastic—Popular works. 2. Women—Surgery. I. Ganny,
    Charlee. II. Title.

RD119.C64 2000
617.9'5'082—dc21   99-049561

10 9 8 7 6 5 4 3 2 1

Design by Tanya Maiboroda
Illustrations by Cathy Pavia
All black-and-white photos and color photo of Charlee Ganny and Susan J. Collini by
Wilton S. Tifft, © 1999. All other photos courtesy of Francis J. Collini.

Published by Renaissance Books
Distributed by St. Martin's Press
Manufactured in the United States of America
First Edition

To my great kids, Lauren and Joey,
and to my especially talented husband, Frank.
Thanks for helping me fulfill my dreams. It's a wonderful life.

—SUSAN

To my sister, Corrine Boland, my best girlfriend,
who said I needed to write down my experiences.
And to the girlfriends at the Renaissance Center—
particularly Barb Gresh, Julie Frederick, and Karen Basar—
whose enthusiasm kept me going.

—CHARLEE

Contents

FOREWORD

I love my profession, and I deeply respect the women who come to me for a plastic-surgery procedure. Both those factors are behind my involvement with this book. Let me tell you how it all started.

The year was 1975, and I had finished my first year at Columbia University in New York City. I registered as a pre-med student, mainly because my dad was an internist and my mother was a nurse. I had nothing planned for the summer so my dad suggested that I volunteer at the Brooklyn Cumberland Hospital where he worked as an attending physician. "Volunteer to do what?" I asked him. He said, "For whatever they need you to do." I figured that if medicine was going to be my future profession, I might as well get my feet wet and see if I liked it. Besides, I had nothing better to do.

The woman at the volunteer office didn't know what to do with me. I was overqualified to be a candy striper, and I didn't want to work in the snack shop. After searching her files, she finally lifted her head and said, "How about the OR?"

My first response was, "They'd let *me* in the operating room?!" The woman at the volunteer office explained that as an orderly I would have full access to the operating room. I jumped at the opportunity.

I was a naive 18-year-old kid from Brooklyn who knew nothing about surgery. There were no surgeons in my family. I had never even met a surgeon. My only exposure to surgery was on TV.

Nevertheless, I was drawn to the OR right from the start. Eventually I befriended the surgeons who worked at the hospital, and they finally allowed me to watch their surgical procedures. I became a learning sponge, soaking up as much knowledge as I could. I had become hooked. Every day when I came home, I described to my parents the operations I had seen. I volunteered my time for the next two summers. I could not get enough.

One day an energetic man arrived in the OR, and I was told he was the attending plastic surgeon. He looked like a movie star, and I was fascinated not only by his surgical skills, but by his persona. He just seemed to have it all, and I wanted to be just like him. The day I watched him do a face-lift is the day plastic surgery became my ultimate goal. I could not believe my eyes as he literally peeled the skin off a woman's face, lifted it, cut it, and then stitched it back together perfectly. The woman looked beautiful when he was done. For years I told everyone who would listen about the surgical details of that face-lift. Now I see face-lifts through different, more educated eyes, but that early fascination with plastic surgery has stayed with me.

Then there was medical school at Downstate in Brooklyn and seven and a half years of surgical residency. The first two years were spent at Johns Hopkins, and the last two at the Mayo Clinic where I learned the art of plastic surgery. It was at Johns Hopkins that I met Susan. She was working as an X-ray technician and at the same time, she was in school to become an ultrasonographer. She was and still is the most beautiful woman I have ever met, both inside and out. We formed a bond that has never broken. She is my partner in business, marriage, and life and we make it work by way of truth, trust, and honesty.

The greatest influence on me as a plastic surgeon was Dr. Richard Ellenbogen, with whom I spent my fellowship in aesthetic surgery in Beverly Hills, California. He was my mentor and a close personal friend who shared with me all of his "secrets." Not only did he teach me to operate, he taught me how to run an office, treat patients, interact with staff, and build a successful practice. I jokingly say, "I am the Ellenbogen of the East Coast."

We all need mentors, idols, heroes to look up to, emulate, and give us drive. We all have stories, and you have just heard mine. Each person who chooses to have plastic surgery has an individual story. As I walk into the consulting room, meeting a patient for the first time, I usually ask, "Have you been thinking about this for a while?" Then I listen. Invariably the patients will proceed to share their personal story with me. Their words usually shed light on their motivation. As their physicians, I want to know who they are, where they are coming from, and where they want to go. I also want to know if I can deliver what they truly want, and moreover, if surgery is what they really need.

About five years ago, Charlee Ganny arrived in my office for her first consultation. She was recently divorced and looking for a "new life." Plastic surgery seemed to be the springboard for her. I listened to her story. We connected, and three surgeries later, she had become, and still is, a beautiful, vivacious woman. The surgery allowed Charlee to look the same way that she felt—young, healthy, happy, and beautiful. You'll hear her story in the pages of this book.

Two Girlfriends Get Real About Plastic Surgery is long overdue in the plastic-surgery world. This book gives a new slant on things and discusses aspects of surgery others don't speak about. Let's face it, 90 percent of plastic-surgical procedures are done on *women,* yet 90 percent of plastic surgeons are *men.* Given this mix, communication is bound to be lacking on certain levels, and patient dissatisfaction most frequently stems from unrealistic expectations and poor preoperative preparation. As a plastic surgeon, I can eloquently describe the nature of a surgical procedure, its risks, benefits, recovery period, and expected outcome. However, I am not very adept at describing how to urinate while wearing a liposuction garment without getting it wet, or how to respond to the problem of envious friends. This book describes things like that, and much more. It uses friendly language and provides a distinct, woman-to-woman perspective. This book bridges the gap between doctor and patient, and allows a woman considering surgery to realize that she is not alone in her questions and fears. This book provides the information needed to allow a woman to make the right decision for herself, and in the process, introduces her to two compassionate, caring, and very outspoken girlfriends.

—*Francis J. Collini, M.D., F.A.C.S.*

Susan's Preface

As women, our bodies are our sanctuaries. They are homes for our confidence, our fear, our peace, and our turmoil. But a woman's body is both public and private. Often these two aspects conflict, and a woman no longer feels comfortable with her self-image, so a change is needed. These changes, however, can be quite frightening. There is a fear of the medical unknown and a fear of the societal myths and secrets involved with cosmetic surgery.

My wish is to help women who are contemplating this life change by helping them dispel the anxiety and reservations associated with surgery. I have spent time with thousands of patients over the past five years, as I've worked side by side with my husband and plastic surgeon, Francis J. Collini, M.D., F.A.C.S. Our practice, the Renaissance Center, includes a certified ambulatory facility with its own operating room and extended recovery-room suite, affiliated day spa, and clothing boutique. It is an environment created for feeling good through the process of maintaining and enhancing one's appearance under qualified supervision. It's a place where many women congregate to share their surgical experiences or to seek "girlfriend info" for potential candidates.

As business manager and patient liaison, I have access to and knowledge of multiple aspects of the Renaissance Center. Furthermore, having undergone several cosmetic surgeries myself, and having a medical background, I am familiar with all of the surgical procedures, recovery times and expectations. My own experiences also permit me to listen empathetically, quelling fears, while providing moral and professional support.

My role also prepares me to advise patients in the areas of insurance, medical costs, hospital operating-room and admission protocols, and doctor/referral relationships and consultations. Listening to and guiding the cosmetic-surgery patient through the vast maze of do's and don'ts, and explaining what one should expect from the first appointment until the last visit, is simplified by my own knowledge and experiences provided by observing our many patients.

When the idea of creating a book was proposed to me by Charlee, I met the challenge with a rush of excitement. From my experiences, I know that every woman contemplating plastic surgery has numerous secret questions, fears, and hopes regarding her pending procedure. Thus, it is my chance to take you by the hand, to educate, dispel myths, and give you the nitty-gritty about what to expect from your surgery. It need not be a mystery anymore.

—*Susan J. Collini, Shavertown, Pennsylvania*

CHARLEE'S PREFACE

You are about to meet some wonderful women in this book, the girlfriends who shared their secrets with Susan and me. I want you to know that each of them is a real person, not a composite. Their stories are true, not fictional. Some girlfriends asked me to change their names, and picked the ones you will know them by. Some, like Denise and Barb, insisted you know their real names, and so I have honored their requests. And by telling all their stories as accurately as I can, I have tried to honor all the girlfriends who dared tell their secrets.

When I started this book, I didn't really know what to expect when I set out to interview the women who had agreed to talk with me about cosmetic surgery. Often I was invited into their homes or office; other times we met in a coffee shop or restaurant. I would find myself standing in the places for "ladies who lunch"—from the best bagel nooks, to espresso bars in bookstores—searching faces, hoping I would walk up and introduce myself to the right woman. Before long I could easily spot the girlfriend by sight, even though I had never met her before. Not one of my girlfriends looked alike, and their ages ranged from in their teens to being in their seventies, but every one of them had a pride in their appearance that was unmistakable. She always stood out from everyone else. Her shoulders were back, her head was high, and she had a presence that made people notice her. She was always well-groomed, whether she was wearing jeans or a business suit. She smelled good, too. I remember the soft perfumes as we drew near to shake hands, or the scent of fresh-washed hair when we hugged to say good-bye. Every girlfriend cared about her looks, and it showed. But there was something else—every girlfriend was smiling.

Shirley Temple's mother told her before she went onstage, "Now, sparkle."

All of the girlfriends sparkled.

All of them had secrets to tell me. And I told them mine.

I liked every single one of them, and I think you will too.

I learned one more thing. These girlfriends are women of incredible courage and independence. They are survivors, fighters, trailblazers. They are women who feel things intensely, so filled with emotion that it often came spilling out when they spoke to me, in laughter, and tears.

They have become my heroes.

Every single one of them was, is, beautiful.

This book is one they wanted written, and one they helped write. They asked me to be honest and not hold back. I haven't. I've told it all as close to the bone as words will let me.

Now, girlfriends, this one's for you . . .

—*Charlee Ganny, on her mountainside in*
Harvey's Lake, Pennsylvania

THE TEN BIGGEST LIES
WOMEN TELL THEMSELVES

1. "I like having small breasts."

2. "I don't look my age."

3. "I don't mind looking like my mother."

4. "This nose gives my face character."

5. "I earned these wrinkles and am damn proud of them."

6. "I'll lose ten pounds—after the holidays."

7. "Makeup can hide the bags under my eyes . . . the scar on my cheek . . . the mole by my nose . . . the lines around my mouth . . ."

8. "My husband loves the way I look."

9. "I *can* flatten my tummy; I just need to start going to the gym."

10. "With the right clothes, nobody notices . . . my thunder thighs . . . my bubble butt . . . my midriff bulge . . . my bingo arms . . . my chicken neck . . ."

INTRODUCTION

Secrets. All women have them. Secrets about sex and men. About money hidden or overspent. About abortions. About a parent who drinks too much. About a family member in prison. About a friend having an affair.

And all women have secrets about their bodies.

What do you think when you look in the mirror? What do you want to hide? Is there some flaw that you have tried to ignore, camouflage, or deny since adolescence or even earlier? What would you change if someone could say a magic spell and make it happen?

"Get the wide-angle lens for Cindy's nose!" her three older brothers would tease every time the camera came out for a photo. They were just kidding, right? So why did the hurt go so deep and stay there?

"Bubble butt!" The words spoken by a fourth-grade classmate haunted Teresa who was stick-thin everywhere except for her high, full derriere.

"I got the 'Fink shelf,'" Sheri moaned, about the family trait of hips that jutted out so far from her torso one could balance a beer tray on them.

Sometimes we do let others know how we feel, but revealing our feelings makes us vulnerable. If we let slip that it bothers us the way our breasts have sagged after having children, someday it might be carelessly, or cruelly, used against us. We are cautious and not trusting. We've learned the hard way about telling secrets, so mostly we hide them inside.

Even today, in our "tell-all" society, most women won't admit they've had cosmetic surgery. The exception may be in southern California, the body-beautiful West Coast, where the latest nip and tuck is a status symbol. But it's still news in the tabloids when a celebrity goes under the knife.

In cosmopolitan New York City, an undercurrent of disapproval ripples through the conversation when the topic is raised, especially among younger women. "Ecch, I'd *never* do that," one twenty-something book editor said about a face-lift. "Never," dear girlfriends, is a very long time, especially when turning forty is very far away. When it's close at hand, or long gone, it's a whole different perspective.

Daisy, an Indiana beauty, came five hundred miles East for a dermabrasion and kept this procedure hidden from everyone except her husband. From what we've seen—in the Midwest, at least—surgery for aesthetic reasons is taboo. In fact, across America in 1998, just 37.6 percent of women admitted they approved of cosmetic surgery for themselves and others, according to a survey by the American Society of Plastic Surgeons (ASPS). The age group with the highest approval rating were women between the ages of 45 and 54, and women with incomes of over $50,000 a year.

Of course women everywhere in the United States *are* doing it. They just keep it secret. How many women actually are having cosmetic surgery? In 1998 nearly three million had surgery, chemical peels, varicose-vein treatments, and Botox injections, according to the ASPS.

But is a cosmetic-surgery procedure right for you? How can you know? Who can you talk to?

One way to find answers is to talk to other women about it.

That's why we wrote this book. Women need to support other women in the decisions they make about their bodies, and they need to share their experiences. Only if we reach out to each other and tell the truth can we make informed, enlightened decisions about what is best for us—even when that truth doesn't fit the "shoulds" that our families, husbands, ethnic backgrounds, shrinks, and our conflict-laden society put on us.

We—Susan and Charlee—learned this by life experience. Both of us were extremely open about our surgeries. Charlee told *everyone:* her manicurist, personal trainer, colleagues, the check-out girl in the supermarket ... Soon women started asking her questions. Many of them had never before spoken out loud their hopes that maybe cosmetic surgery could help them. They asked about more than the surgery itself. They wanted to know how to pay for a procedure, how to find the best surgeon, how to squeeze surgery in with work and family schedules, how to hide the fact they had had it, how to reduce their risks and avoid complications ... and how—oh, how!—did they get over being scared? Most of them were "scared shitless!" Charlee says, sitting in her home office surrounded by her computers, books, and her three dogs and ten cats.

Susan, sitting in a very different location, had been talking to prospective clients of her husband's for five years. The women she met in the office setting were at a different stage than the women who talked to Charlee, since these girlfriends had gone beyond merely thinking about cosmetic surgery—they had taken steps to have a consultation with a surgeon. Even so, most of them admitted that talking about their bodies was difficult; talking about their feelings was even more so. Only when Susan revealed her own experiences, opening up her private self and speaking personally, did women risk exposing the concerns, hurts, and fears hidden inside them.

Between them, Charlee and Susan were talking to scores of women—and finally Charlee and Susan started talking to each other and decided to work together on a book so they could bring information and support about plastic surgery from the patient's point of view to women everywhere.

So here, in the pages that follow, are real girlfriends, real experiences, and frank talk about cosmetic surgery. Cosmetic surgery is *not* right for everyone. Some procedures are a lot riskier than others. There are always trade-offs, no matter what procedure a woman chooses, whether it is the long scar of a tummy tuck, or the fat that comes back in weird places after liposuction.

We give you the straight scoop. We don't pretty-up anything. We talk flat-out about "taboo" subjects, from having to pee and poop after a butt tuck, to sex positions after breast augmentation. Maybe for the first time in a book, we discuss some body secrets women still keep hidden: One example is what pregnancy can really do to your body, and another is the best-kept lie about the consequences of dieting and weight loss.

But we also ask you to do something, too: Take full responsibility for the decisions you make, and act as an equal partner in your surgery. We will provide you with compassion, understanding, support, and the most useful tool of empowerment—knowledge. And girlfriend, ain't nobody going to do more for you than that. In this life, you have to do for yourself. *You* must take care of yourself. *You* have to do the work of finding a good doctor. *You* have to spill your guts to your doctor about drug and alcohol use, eating disorders, and pill taking—or risk losing your life. *You* have to get over the embarrassment of discussing the size of your breasts or the shape of your nose. *You* have to have the courage and bear the pain. *You* have to put yourself *first* after surgery: Give yourself permission to have the care, the time, and the right to recover fully without getting out of bed to wash clothes the day after surgery, run the vacuum, or sneak into the office.

And we will tell you over and over: Plastic surgery is something you do for yourself. Only for yourself. It is altering your body forever. No one has the right to do that—or control that—but you. No one should urge you to do it. *But no one has the right to stop you from doing it.*

For many women, getting plastic surgery becomes the first step toward autonomy and real independence. For some, it lets the genie out of the bottle, and there's no way to put it back. The toothpaste is out of the tube.

The debate may still go on among the psychiatric profession about the motives for and consequences of plastic surgery, but we have seen real life. When women feel good about themselves, they get stronger. They get more assertive. They become a force that says, "Look out, world." The men in their life are either thrilled . . . or out the door. That's the truth. Plastic surgery changes more than the body. If you aren't ready for emotional changes or life changes, you aren't ready for surgery. If you've already begun developing a healthy lifestyle, focusing on self-care, and handling reality in a positive way, surgery can be another step for reaching the goals you've been dreaming about—or a catalyst for making important career or relationship changes.

One final note: We cover many cosmetic-surgery procedures, more than you will probably find anywhere else, but we haven't tried to cover all of them. We give you the latest information available at this time. But new techniques are being developed daily; medicines and lotions and machines and "breakthroughs" in anti-aging treatments are happening all the time. We ask you to investigate everything! We can examine what exists now. Most procedures won't change much, like nose jobs, "the oldest procedure." But for the "latest" in plastic surgery, go to the library! Update what we tell you before you get pumped up, sucked, nipped, or tucked.

How to Use This Book

We have organized this book in two distinct parts. The first part, sections 1–4, covers specific cosmetic surgeries one by one; the second part, section 5, gives you information you need only after you decide to have surgery.

Each section in the first part of the book covers the most popular procedures being done today. The chapters are organized according to the location of the "problem" with appearance. You can read the chapters that relate to your concerns, or browse through the entire book, even if you just want to read the true-life stories of all the girlfriends who spoke with us. Here is a quick synopsis of what you will find:

In chapter 1 Susan and Charlee tell you what catalysts—a life event or an inner crisis—move many women to decide to have cosmetic surgery. Some fun self-tests will help you clarify your own thinking and make a decision, too. And there are provocative questions to help you examine *why* you want surgery and what psychologists say about the women who have made this choice. You may be very surprised at their conclusions.

Next is section 1, which includes chapters 2, 3, and 4. This section addresses women's number one concern about their appearance—and the leading reason they choose cosmetic surgery. No, it's not aging. It's FAT.

Chapter 2 carefully reviews today's most popular cosmetic-surgery procedure, liposuction. You will find out what liposuction actually is, what happens to you when you have it, and where it works well on your body—and where it doesn't! Finally you'll be warned about the shocking consequences of any weight gain *after* the procedure . . . and how you could end up with a big fat problem in places you never dreamed you could add inches.

Chapter 3 provides everything you need to know about one of the most serious cosmetic-surgery operations—the tummy tuck, or abdominoplasty. This operation has its drawbacks to be sure—but it is the procedure with the most dramatic results. For some women, it can literally erase years of shame and discomfort, particularly if that girlfriend is enduring the physical aftereffects of pregnancy nobody talks about. It's called post-pregnancy syndrome, and it's a heartbreaker. But a tummy tuck will heal a broken heart . . . and create a beautiful body too.

Chapter 4 reveals an area of plastic surgery most women don't even know exists: skin reduction, or body contouring. These procedures—and they include belt abdominoplasty, buttock tuck, thighplasty, and more—are the only way to rejuvenate a body gone south; in other words, taking a fifty-year-old butt and making it look fifteen again. These surgeries are the *only* way to get rid of the bumps and lumps of cellulite—no matter what you've heard about creams, massages, or even liposuction. They are also the only way to deal with the dirtiest little secret of weight loss: excess skin. The weight is gone, the fat is gone, but baggy, saggy, hideous skin remains . . . until a woman goes under the knife. Are the results miraculous? They certainly can be. Are there trade-offs? You bet your bippie . . . and your scars.

Section 2 is all about boobs. Chapter 5 gives you the nitty-gritty on breast implants, the second-most-popular cosmetic surgery procedure, and the one most younger women undergo. Why are they doing it? In this chapter girlfriends speak out, bluntly, about their motives. Take the case of one girlfriend who encountered a loud objection from her male personal trainer about her upcoming breast augmentation surgery: "Why would you want to do that to yourself?" he screamed. "I can't understand it. You have a great body the way you are!" With great dignity, she pulled herself up tall, looked him straight in the eye, and said, "If you could add two inches to your penis, would you do it?" End of discussion. But are implants safe? Will a new lover know you had it done . . . and should you reveal the truth? Which size or shape implant is best? Chapter 5 handles the boob controversy by providing essential facts—plus lots of laughs.

Chapter 6 examines the other side of the coin: women who have too much and want less! A well-endowed girlfriend whose family originally came from southern Italy—home of many big-breasted women, including Neapolitan beauty Sophia Loren—confessed she had been miserable because of the size of her breasts *since she was ten years old.* She chose to wear blazers and loose tops to disguise her full figure. She had never found a comfortable bra. She looked pounds heavier than she actually was. She *hated* the way she looked. For this girlfriend and all her compadres, chapter 6 holds great news about new techniques and fabulous results.

Section 3 covers what most people think about when they hear the term "cosmetic surgery." Chapter 7 deals with face-lifts, which younger and younger women are undergoing each year. A procedure that is usually painless (most women don't know that!), a good face-and-neck–lift wipes away decades overnight. This surgery can produce results that are truly miraculous, and, performed by a good surgeon, it is amazingly safe. For many women, the astonishing results can save their sanity, their self-esteem, spark a new relationship, or change their employment outlook. Chapter 7 tells all!

Chapter 8 takes women into unknown territory, or, at least, unknown to the general public. These are the procedures that can be done along with a face-lift, or on their own, to rejuvenate a woman's appearance, eliminate a disfigurement, or make an ordinary woman gorgeous. Is that just hype? No, ma'am. It's just the plain truth. For example, find out about "witch's chin"—another unpleasant aspect of aging—and how to fix it so you look like a princess. Discover how easy it is to have a model's high cheekbones, to improve a profile, or to make tired eyes look vibrant. It's all here.

Chapter 9 explores the operation that might be the most emotionally loaded of all the procedures: nose jobs. A woman's relationship to her nose goes deep—especially if she hates it. Often the root of self-esteem issues since childhood, a large or misshapen nose has undoubtedly exposed a woman to teasing and trauma at home and in school. Is a rhinoplasty the answer? At what age? How successful is the operation? What are the dangers? Are women happy afterward? Why do many of them experience an overwhelming sense of loss? Chapter 9 sensitively and compassionately talks about why a nose is a nose is a nose.

Section 4 gives it to you straight on wrinkles. Chapter 10 talks frankly about the hottest new procedure, laser resurfacing. It's a serious procedure where a woman can get burned—and it's where Susan and Charlee take perhaps their most controversial stand. Yes, it can leave skin looking like Devonshire cream or the finest porcelain. But, oh baby, it can be a disaster. Read Susan's personal story about her laser ordeal and find out what you need to know!

Chapter 11 gives women an alternative to laser treatments, the old stand-by, dermabrasion. Long used to help smooth out disfiguring acne scars, dermabrasion may be a wise choice for resurfacing, but this "wounding" of the skin has its drawbacks, too. And what about the new Parisian peels, those quickie, lunchtime treatments that are really light dermabrasion treatments? Should you spend your money? We give you firsthand reports.

Chapter 12 reviews the chemical peels, and we tell you the continuing good news about Retin-A and the exciting news about Botox. Increasing numbers of women are having Botox, a "temporary" wrinkle remover, injected into areas of their face. How long does it last? How well does it work? Has it given collagen and fat injections a shove out the door? Here are the surprising facts on Botox—and some promising reports on AlloDerm, the latest "filler" for facial lines.

The second part of the book, section 5, covers information that is essential to every woman who is seriously considering a specific procedure or has made plans to undergo surgery. Developed from the input of real-life women who are veterans of plastic surgery, it helps you prepare for surgery and recover safely. And it tells you what other books don't: how to cope socially and emotionally with the results.

Chapter 13 guides you in your search to find the best possible plastic surgeon. It explains how to follow a paper trail to hunt down a qualified doctor, what questions to ask during a consultation, recommends the use of a girlfriend-advocate, and helps you evaluate both the doctor and the surgical facility. This chapter puts aside the humor to deal head-on with the precautions that may save your life.

Chapter 14 gets to the bottom line. Surgery costs money—often very big bucks. But most of the women who are flocking into clinics and doctors' offices aren't rich. A large percentage of them are working women who deal with the public: beauticians, nurses, sales personnel, teachers, and independent business owners; a number of them are young, hopeful, but often broke exotic dancers, aspiring actresses, and struggling models. Where does the money come from? Here are suggestions, stories, and outrageous antics for coming up with the cash.

Chapter 15 is the chapter a surgery candidate needs to read like the Bible. It's the one to photocopy and carry around in your purse. It spells out what you need to do to prepare, emotionally and physically, for surgery. It tells you what real-life women have found out, and what insider tips can get you in peak condition to sail through surgery with a minimum of discomfort and complications. Then Susan and Charlee give you sound, authoritative advice on what to do *after* surgery: Here are the general do's and don'ts that help you recovery safely and quickly from any surgery.

Chapter 16 is a hoot. It shares girlfriends' advice about who to tell and what to say. Even if you decide to be totally honest about your surgery, the consensus is, there are some people you should never tell. You will find a treasure house of girlfriends' very best lies, most ingenious fibs, and absolutely wonderful confabulations to use as you need them.

Chapter 17 is the grand finale, a short look at lives transformed by surgery. What are the social and emotional consequences of changing the way you look? We tell the whole story of one very special transformation.

You can read this book cover to cover and not be bored. But most likely you will zero in on the section covering the procedure you've been considering. You'll get your questions answered, and the facts you need to decide what choices are right for you. One thing we promise you, in this book, you will be among friends.

The Moment of Truth: Deciding to Have Plastic Surgery

No woman wakes up one morning and decides to have plastic surgery. For a long time a voice in your head has been saying, *I hate . . . my nose . . . the way my belly looks after having kids . . . the jowls that are forming along my chin line.* The idea of surgery comes to you and stays with you. But it usually takes a long time before you do anything about it. The reasons may be financial, but mostly you are wrestling with deeper questions. *Am I being vain? Shouldn't I accept myself as I am? Will my husband approve? What if the surgery doesn't turn out? Should I take the risk? Can surgery really help me, or am I fantasizing?*

Almost all the women we talked to had thought about surgery for a long time, and had changed their minds more than once. Some girlfriends had already begun improving their body image by dieting and going to the gym, and growing emotionally by working on their lives. Cosmetic surgery seemed like a natural next step for women like Anne:

> My surgery was part of a complete program of taking care
> of myself. I weighed over 200 pounds after my son was born.
> I would mope around the house all day in sweatpants,

and really felt bad about myself. Finally I got myself together and began to lose weight. When I got down to about 160 I started going to the gym three times a week. I still do: That's time for me to take care of me. I had spent most of my younger life putting everyone else first—and it just doesn't work in the long run.

Most women ponder their decision. Other women, like Barb Gresh, have an epiphany, a moment when they just know they are going to do it. But for many girlfriends, the decision to have surgery emerges from a life crisis. Here are some of the most common events that propel a woman into the surgeon's office.

Breast Cancer and Plastic Surgery

A surprising number of girlfriends we talked with decided to have an aesthetic plastic surgery procedure after a mastectomy. This sequence of events really makes perfect sense. Breast reconstruction often brings a woman into a plastic surgeon's office for the first time. She meets and gets to like a doctor, so the next step—having a consultation about another procedure—is easy.

On a psychological level, a woman with breast cancer has had a brush with death. Before this confrontation with mortality she may have been putting off doing things for herself, always considering the needs of her husband and children first. Her illness makes her realize she needs time for herself. Her plastic surgery is as important an expense as her husband's new set of golf clubs—and perhaps a lot more essential. Sometimes a cancer survivor looks in the mirror and sees the anxiety, fears, and strain of her illness on her face and body. Now, by having a face-lift, liposuction, or other surgery, she can look at her reflection and see a vibrant, healthy, and alive woman. The results boost her self-esteem and make her feel good about the way she looks. They also affirm to herself—and the world—that she has survived!

R.I.P—Death and Cosmetic surgery

The death of a significant other, or a family member or friend, often provides a similar catalyst for girlfriends deciding it is time for cosmetic surgery. Improving their physical appearance is a proclamation of life, a denial of death and aging, as if a woman is saying, "Someone I loved is dead, but *I'm* not dying. *I'm* alive." Often, if she was the caregiver, she feels she can now focus on herself. For grieving girlfriends, rejuvenating their appearance is part of the healing process, a way of going on with life, a new beginning.

Other widowed women have this thought: "Now there's no one to stop me from having cosmetic surgery." The person who opposed or disapproved of a surgery no longer stands in the way.

D-I-V-O-R-C-E and Cosmetic Surgery

Breaking up with a man is another event that spurs some women to get cosmetic surgery. Some hurt, angry women want to show the ex just what he lost and make him eat his heart out. Others think they can get him back by looking so good he can't resist. Raquel, whose longtime husband left her for a younger woman, admitted this was in the back of her mind. Interestingly, Raquel is extremely attractive, but said to us she didn't feel she was. She said she had difficulty developing a new relationship. She felt unable to sever her ties with her ex, who, frankly, was playing head games with her; breaking down crying in front of her and sobbing that he couldn't bear to think about what had happened to her. He called her daily. He stopped in for dinner several times a week—before leaving to go back to his new fiancée's bed.

Girlfriends, does this scenario sound all too familiar? Surgery gave Raquel a beautiful face—but she hadn't internalized the change. She was still missing the energy and self-confidence that

"What was the moment when I decided to have surgery? I was on a romantic cruise through the Greek islands with my husband. The sky was intensely blue; the sun was scorching. I put on a bathing suit, and suddenly I just couldn't take how I looked anymore. My waist was 21 inches, my upper body was a size 4—and my hips, thighs, and legs were a size 16. I was completely out of proportion. There had not been a day of my adult life that I had felt good about my body. Now I was thirty-seven years old. I remembered a story on 20/20 about new liposuction techniques. Right then, I knew I was going to do it."

BARB GRESH

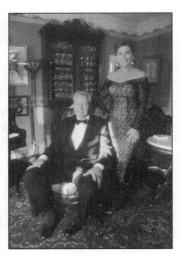

Barb Gresh poses with her husband after lower-body reduction surgeries (liposuction, thighplasty, butt tuck, and abdominoplasty). She wore a teensy weensy bikini on her last cruise and looked fabulous.

make men come buzzing around for a look. Honey, you don't need a face-lift to project the most irresistible quality in the world. It's called charisma! It comes entirely from within.

So when it comes to an ex, forget about using cosmetic surgery to win him back. Move on with your life! If you really want him to come back, you have to *not* want him. Only when you are not "needy," only when you are seeing others and having a great time, will he come crawling back to your door. Otherwise he'll keep you dangling for years . . . for a lifetime. Our advice? Find someone who thinks you're the grand prize, not the second runner-up. Remember the wise old saying, "Living well is the best revenge."

However, *can* surgery help a woman compete in the dating game and attract a new partner? Yes. Looking terrific—and projecting that you look terrific—will get you dates. It won't earn you love, and it won't help you keep a relationship going. But to be honest, girlfriends, looking gorgeous makes it a whole lot easier to be choosy and not act desperate. Yes, girlfriends, cosmetic surgery can help mend a broken heart. Here's a true story:

Pixie-faced Pauline was headed for the big four-oh and was busy with her journalism career. She had been with her longtime steady, Rob, a businessman, for eight years. Both of them had jobs that kept them traveling, and they were used to spending a lot of time apart. Pauline expected they would get married after Rob finally sold his family's company, something that had been in the works for a while. Once that happened, he promised, he would give serious thought to tying the knot.

When Rob finally went out of town to finish up the company's sale, Pauline gave him a peck on the cheek and a cheery, "I'll see you when you get back." Rob sent her a card from another city and he called, but more often than not, they played telephone tag on their answering machines. Weeks went by. Then the phone calls stopped. Pauline didn't hear a word. Busy, working on a major story, she blew it off. She figured Rob needed some space; after all, this sale would change his life.

Three months had passed when she started to panic. She hadn't heard from Rob for . . . she couldn't even remember when they talked last. A lonely Friday night, a glass of wine, and an old movie set off an anxiety attack. Pauline decided to track Rob down. She called his hotel. He'd checked out weeks ago. She called his apartment. The number was disconnected. Finally, at nine o'clock at night, she called the company that had been for sale. No one picked up the phone, but she let it ring and ring and ring and ring. Miracle of miracles, someone finally answered—someone she actually knew.

"Oh, hi, Pauline! Rob? Yep, he finished up handing everything over to the new owners and he just left today," his former VP said. "Sure I know where he is; he's staying with his brother."

Blessed relief flooded through Pauline. She knew Rob's brother. She had his telephone number. She dialed. "Hi, Ben, this is Pauline. Is Rob there?" There was an awkward silence; then, "Oh, hi, Pauline. No, um, Rob isn't here."

"Where is he? I haven't heard from him in weeks!"

"Um, Pauline, I guess he didn't tell you. Rob met somebody."

" 'Met somebody'? What do you mean?"

"I mean— Well, I'm sorry, but Rob's engaged. He's getting married in two weeks. He went to Cleveland to close the company sale and met a girl he went with in high school. It was sudden, you know. They just clicked. I'm sorry, Pauline. He should have told you."

The next day Pauline went in for a consultation for full-face laser surgery. She took ten years off her looks, has a face as smooth, soft, and wrinkle-free as a baby's bottom, and figures she looks two years younger than she did when she first met Rob. Then she started dating with a vengeance. There is a happy ending, girlfriends. Pauline met a new guy, and she's slowed down on her career track and speeded up on the love line.

> **LEGAL DETAIL**
>
> **A** note for soon-to-be ex-wives: Some divorced girlfriends negotiated to include the price of their cosmetic surgery in their divorce settlement. That made the whole experience so much sweeter.

But I'm thinking about plastic surgery, and I didn't have
a life crisis . . . Do I have some deep-seated problem?

Psychiatrists used to have a field day with women who opted for plastic surgery, and male patients, the poor dears, really got slammed. In fact, the prevailing wisdom twenty years ago advised plastic surgeons that a male patient who wanted the procedure was neurotic, or worse! But new studies are showing something very different about both men and women who opt for surgery; they report that women who have plastic-surgery procedures have more of their self-esteem invested in their appearance than women who don't. They spend more time and energy with personal grooming, consider themselves physically attractive, and are more satisfied with their overall body image than other women (Sarwer, 231). Translated into everyday English, the psychological mumbo-jumbo means: If you're a good-looking woman, chances are you are going to invest time, energy, and money into staying that way.

Susan Collini, for one, undergoes "grilling" by some of her friends about why she feels the need to "maintain" her beauty through cosmetic surgery. They ask her, why can't she accept herself? Does she have to be perfect? One has even suggested she needs to examine herself for deep-seated psychological issues. Be aware, girlfriends, you could be asked these questions, too. Keep in mind that jealousy may be at work here, even on an unconscious level, because women are so competitive with one another. But taking these inquiries as expressions of concern, let us reassure others that working women, especially women working in the "beauty" industry, need to look well-groomed and attractive. Susan runs a day spa, manages a plastic-surgery corporation, and is the owner-buyer for her clothing boutique. If she herself hadn't had some of the procedures women consult her about, where would her credibility be? If she didn't believe in the surgeries' value, where would her honesty be? Since she is intelligent, physically healthy, a successful businesswoman, a talented interior decorator, a loving wife and mother with two good kids, upbeat, fun, and compassionate (plus she doesn't drink, smoke, or take drugs), where are the signs of neurosis, psychosis, or abnormality in her behavior? What issues are interfering in her ability to function and succeed? Give us a break! Pull in the claws!

If you are thinking about plastic surgery, you probably have a reason to want to improve your appearance—and are tired of throwing away money on products that promise help, but deliver only disappointment. Psychological testing has shown there's nothing wrong with your self-esteem if you opt for plastic surgery; it falls well within normal ranges (Terino, 11). And if it's your nose that you wish to change, studies have also shown that your perception is accurate: In other words, other people notice it, too. Are you wrong for wanting to remove a disfigurement or to be prettier? If wanting to be more attractive were a true personality flaw, the cosmetic industry would go bankrupt.

Despite all the spiritual and psychological advice we hear to "accept" ourselves, love our bodies, build up the inner person, our culture gives us an entirely different message in much bigger doses. Don't mistake what we're saying here; we're not saying this is a good situation. But it is reality. Our culture favors attractive people, discounts the value of older workers in the workplace, and idealizes a strong, athletic, slim body. And given a choice, most people would opt to look healthy, attractive, young, and energetic; perhaps human beings have always preferred that—so why are women wrong to aspire to it? But today in America, certain means of improvements are acceptable, including hair dye, makeup, capped teeth, contact lenses, manicures and artificial nails, working out to tone and firm the body, anti-aging medications, push-up bras, minimizer undergarments . . . Yet one method that significantly improves one's appearance ain't kosher: cosmetic surgery. Go figure.

"If the body is a temple, should we not adorn it?"

GLORIA, HOSPITAL NURSE

You're getting older . . . and you're getting better.

Not one girlfriend we met wanted to be young again. Every single one of them valued their age, wisdom, and life experiences. But no one wanted the negative changes age had brought to their figure and skin. In fact, there's nothing positive about *physical* aging, and our culture still gives us a double standard when it comes to cosmetic surgery.

It is socially acceptable to have surgery to fix a sagging internal organ, to maintain our teeth, or to correct cataracts. We are expected to diet (even though it doesn't work)—in fact, obesity is a sin! No one would advocate contentment with arthritis, osteoporosis, varicose veins, or balding. But when the largest organ on our body, the skin, is damaged by age and environmental factors, we are "going against nature" if we fix it. We must live with sagging skin, wrinkles, jowls, hanging necks, warts, moles, chin hair, discoloration. And if we dare use liposuction or surgery to remove unwanted fat, it's a sacrilege.

Hogwash! Stop the judging. Stop the nonsensical "rules." These attitudes are arbitrary, illogical, and ultimately cruel.

Especially when you reach those milestone birthdays—thirty, forty, fifty, sixty, and seventy—you may find yourself looking closely at the changes in your body and face. We've supplied an objective self-test for determining if you're ready for a face-lift (see pages 129–31), but subjectively you probably have some strong feelings about the signs of aging, environmental damage, inherited abnormalities, or changes caused by childbearing. These feelings are valid. Don't discount them.

Is it time to do something about body or facial "flaws"? Girlfriend Rosemary C. advises a woman to have a procedure done before the physical characteristic becomes a familiar part of her appearance. In other words, if your family is known for large pouches under the eyes, you may be seeing this trait before you turn thirty. If you wait until you are forty to have surgery, people will notice because many of them will never have seen you look any differently. If you do it when the trait first shows (and this is true of jowls, sagging necks, and wrinkles, too), you may look "healthier," "rested," "thinner," but no one will guess you had surgery.

So ask yourself these three questions:

1. Does the change in your appearance brought by time add anything positive to your life?

2. Does it make sense to throw away money on "concealers" that don't real conceal anything or "face-lifts in a jar" that don't work?

3. Is it "vain" to remove the change permanently and restore your original appearance?

You know the answers: No; no; and no! Stop beating yourself up. If it's okay to spend a fortune on makeup to try to cover up the bags under your eyes, why isn't okay to have a lower blepharoplasty (a very safe, not-too-expensive, and almost painless procedure) and forever remove the bags that make you look tired, haggard, and unhealthy?

But aren't some women who have plastic surgery "meshuga"?

There is a psychological disorder that manifests itself as a misperception that something is wrong with your body, or as a hatred of your own body. It's called *dysmorphia*. Here's what the literature says about this mental disorder and plastic surgery:

> These relatively normal-appearing patients misperceive their appearance, they have a subjective feeling of ugliness related to a perceived physical defect less noticeable to others than to themselves (Anderson, 228–29).

So how do you know if you are "misperceiving" something about your body that is bothering you? If you know someone who is plainspoken, somewhat inconsiderate of the feelings of others, and uncomfortably honest, you could ask her.

> Q: "Aunt Blanche, if you had a nose like mine, what would you do?"
>
> A: "Bubbele, I'd wear a paper bag on my head."

If you don't have someone to ask, here are questions to ask yourself. They should help you clarify whether you have a valid concern and would truly benefit from plastic surgery.

BODY IMAGE EVALUATION QUESTIONNAIRE

1. What is it about your body or face that you feel is a flaw (or, if connected to aging, that you see as a negative change)?

   ("Yes" answers to any of the next set of questions indicate you have a valid concern about your body image and have good reasons to want to change it.)

2. Have you been teased by family members and friends about the flaw that concerns you?

3. Do you buy clothes to accommodate the flaw? Are there some articles of clothing or jewelry you will not wear?

4. Are you spending significant money on cosmetic and anti-aging products?

5. Have you ever sent for mail-order or infomercial products designed to improve your appearance? (Products to eliminate or reduce the appearance of acne and acne scars should be included here.)

6. Do you believe the flaw has affected you socially? Do you feel uncomfortable about meeting people? Have you ever refused a job opportunity because of it? Do you feel you were ever overlooked for a job opportunity because of it?

7. Has a significant other ever used this flaw to attack your self-esteem?

8. Has aging or obesity so changed your appearance that you feel you are losing your sexual identity? feel less worthy as a human being? feel inferior to others? feel at a disadvantage in a social setting?

9. Can you clearly describe the change you want?

10. Do you have reasonable expectations from plastic surgery? In other words, if you expect to duplicate a film star's nose or end up with a perfect face, you have unreasonable expectations. If you hope for a 50 to 75 percent improvement in your appearance, but not perfection—and with some negatives from the surgery—you have realistic expectations.

    (*"Yes" to the next set of questions may indicate the need for some psychological support in dealing with your body image.*)

11. Have you had plastic surgery before on the same area . . . more than several times? (If so, you may be dismorphic. If it's like twenty times, you have your answer.)

12. Are you under treatment or medication for anxiety, depression, or a sleep disorder? Do you have a drug or alcohol problem? (If so, you might want to check your perception of your body imperfections with a professional.)

13. Are you in the middle of a life crisis? (If so, you need to wait until the situation is stable or resolved before you make any major decisions—including whether or not to have plastic surgery.)

14. Do you have any concerns regarding gender/sexual identity issues? (Plastic surgery may still be appropriate, but realize your unhappiness with your appearance is also tied to other issues [Anderson, 228].)

"I was a fat baby. I was a fat kid. I was fat all my life. Before my surgery I was 245 pounds. From the very first time I heard about liposuction, it was on my mind that I wanted to do it. I didn't want to be thin. I just wanted a waistline—something I never had. After surgery I put on a size 14 dress with a belt, when I had been an apple-shaped size 22 a few weeks earlier. When I saw how I looked, nothing could stop me from getting more done."

SHERI

Being Honest with Yourself

The bottom line on cosmetic surgery depends entirely on your own degree of satisfaction with your appearance—and your knowledge about what you can do to change it. Maybe you are certain you would change your thighs, breasts, face, nose, or stomach if you could. But you don't know enough about the surgery to make a decision.

If this is your situation, read on. If you are just curious, read on.

By knowing your options, you can make an informed choice about what is best for you.

THE SKINNY ON FAT

2

THE MOST POPULAR PROCEDURE: LIPOSUCTION

Bubble butt, thunder thighs, saddlebags, piano legs, potbelly, spare tire, granny arms, double chin . . . No matter how much we diet or exercise, there are some areas of our body that won't budge except to bulk up further. It's genetic. It's unavoidable. But it is no longer our fate. Now we have liposuction!

The concept of surgical body contouring—i.e., the surgical removal of body fat and skin—has been around since the profession of plastic and reconstructive surgery began. However, until the discovery of liposuction, surgical contouring left your body with a road map of scars. Now, liposuction and newer surgical techniques have vastly reduced the scarring associated with body contouring. Suddenly women are getting sucked and tucked in vast numbers, with liposuction leading the field: 149,042 procedures done in 1998 alone, according to the American Society of Plastic Surgeons.

Liposuction sounds like such a great idea. No more dieting! No more denial! Just get on the table and get your fat sucked out. But there is a catch, isn't there? Of course there is.

What is the catch? What are the trade-offs? That's what girlfriends need to know.

THE ART OF GETTING SUCKED

Lustrous dark hair frames September's smooth, unlined face. She is not model-slim, but tall and well-proportioned. There are no bulges in the wrong places when she wears her crisp white nurse's uniform. Now, her big brown eyes filling with tears, September explains why she had full-body liposuction: a tummy tuck, a buttock tuck, and a thighplasty.

> I had my first child at thirty-seven years old. Seven months after his birth I found a lump on my right breast. A biopsy showed it was malignant. I quickly had a lumpectomy, radiation treatments, and started chemo.

She stops talking because her voice has begun trembling uncontrollably. Six years after her diagnosis the pain and fear still well up and overwhelm her. She waits a minute, to regain her composure, then she continues:

> You can't imagine how it felt to have an infant and face the possibility I might not be there for him. The experience was

I HAVE FAT THIGHS—WHY ME?

Fat distribution on your body is determined by two factors, heredity and diet. Heredity determines the number and location of every fat cell in your body. The *number* of fat cells in your body does not change after puberty, but diet can increase or decrease the *amount* of fat contained in these fat cells. If you inherited more fat cells in your thighs than in other areas of your body, then you will always have more fat on your thighs than other places *no matter how much weight you lose or how long you exercise.*

Once liposuction removes the fat cells from, for example, your thighs, you will not get as fat there again. We used to think you couldn't get fat there at all. Wrong! As long as any cells are left, you can start expanding. But since there are far fewer, if you gain weight after having liposuction, you will get fatter . . . someplace else, someplace unexpected, someplace where you will absolutely hate having fat.

devastating. Then I went into chemo-induced menopause. My weight shot up to over two hundred pounds and stayed there. My breasts enlarged from a B cup to a DD. I am tall, nearly five foot seven. I never weighed more than 155 in my life. I was never fat, never. Now, finding myself obese after the trauma of breast cancer, I fell into a dark, total despair. No amount of dieting or exercise worked. I felt as if my own body kept betraying me.

On the advice of my oncologist I had a breast reduction. That was when I found my plastic surgeon. The surgery turned out beautifully, but the radiated tissue of my right breast refused to heal. Before I knew what was happening I landed in the hospital with a virulent infection in my right breast. My plastic surgeon had to operate again to clean out the irradiated tissue and the infection. As a result of this complication, I was left with a "hollow" or depression on my breast, and it made the size of my breasts uneven, but that was in no way the fault of my plastic surgeon. Women need to know that tissue that has been heavily irradiated just does not heal.

In fact, I felt so much confidence in my surgeon that I asked about surgery to get my body back. We set up a series of procedures to reduce my body fat in stages. Full-body lipo from under my breasts to my knees and a tummy tuck not only salvaged my self-esteem; it may have saved my life.

With a waist that measures no more than 21 inches, blonde, lovely Catherine, at thirty-five, looks exactly like what she is: a professional bodybuilder and model. She has told no one that she, too, has had liposuction. When it comes to secrets, men and women bodybuilders or fitness trainers may have the most carefully hidden ones of all. They often have had liposuction, various types of tucks, and implants in their breasts (women) or pectoral muscles and calves (men)—and they never tell. If you can see those washboard abs, it means there is little or no fat covering them. Where did that fat go? Sometimes it goes down the vacuum tube.

Catherine's figure fault was saddlebags on her outer thighs: "I spend hours every day at the gym. Exercise? Tell me about it," she explained. "I eat 'clean.' I do everything right. Nothing I did budged the fat on my thighs. My body was not at all in proportion. That's why I did liposuction."

What the sucking is all about.

Two kinds of liposuction are currently popular in Europe and the United States: SAL (suction-assisted lipoplasty) and UAL (ultrasound-assisted lipoplasty). The ultrasound procedure received a great deal of media attention a few years ago, but it hasn't lived up to its publicity (see sidebar, page 53). However, ultrasound liposuction has found its niche during long operations where a great deal of fat is removed.

Liposuction surgery can be performed in the physician's office, at an outpatient surgical facility, or in a hospital, depending on the physician's determination of the patient's health and the amount of fat reduction. Liposuction is done using a local anesthetic and intravenous sedation, but a small area can be done with local anesthetic alone.

Most patients are between the ages of sixteen and fifty-five. However, age is not a deterrent, as girlfriends in their sixties can get great results, too; it depends on your overall health and skin elasticity. And if you are very overweight, over 225 pounds, you will face special risks. It doesn't mean you can't have liposuction; in fact, liposuction for obesity is becoming more accepted as an option. But you may be hospitalized for it; you may receive a transfusion of your own blood; and you may have to have liposuction more than once, along with a tummy tuck, a buttock tuck, a thighplasty, and/or a skin reduction procedure.

What parts of the body are appropriate for liposuction contouring? Here is what we found.

- Jowls. Liposuction of the face has a downside. It certainly removes fat, but if there is poor skin tone here, liposuction will make it worse. Best bet to get rid of jowls: Get a face-lift.

- Neck and under the chin. Liposuction on the neck under the chin area can produce very good results. The skin adheres well afterward and the improvement in appearance after removing a "double chin" or making the area more defined can be astonishing (Goddio, 66). Men, for a refreshing change, have more sagging in the skin here than women. But for the best results, liposuction combined with a face-lift will produce a classic, smooth, youthful contour.

- Bulge above the breast, toward your armpit, sticking out of your bra strap. Ugh! The skin is thin; the fat is soft. You will get significant improvement here, but not complete "contraction" (Lillis, 974). If the problem is severe, and you don't mind a scar, you might opt for having the fat cut out along with the excess skin (Collini).

- Bra-line fat bulge (same as above but on your back). The skin is quite thick here and you get good results (Lillis, 974).

- Upper back. Thick skin that generally contracts well, can give terrific results, even for women in their sixties (Fodor and Watson, 1114).

- Lower back. From below your bra strap to your waist, or "water wings"—this is another good site for terrific results (Lillis, 974).

- Waist. The good news is that the skin here almost always contracts back in beautifully, and is one of the most gratifying areas to many girlfriends who have been previously "shapeless." Girlfriend Sheri had thrilling results—and a waist for the first time in her life. Girlfriend, have to tell you, we find this area almost irresistibly tempting!

- Abdomen. The bad news is that your skin is likely to sag here. You will reduce the size of your tummy, but liposuction alone does not produce outstanding results. You may need a tummy tuck.

- Hips. That shelf that is so handy for sitting a child on, but makes clothes that fit impossible to find, also makes us look matronly. Liposuction works very well here (Lillis, 975).

- Upper outer thighs (saddlebags). This is one of the most popular sites for liposuction. It will definitely remove that stubborn fat that just won't disappear even if you start marathon racing. However, there is a downside. Liposuction of the saddlebags may create puckering, indentation, and even a depression. But for some girlfriends, especially if they are thin elsewhere, the results may be spectacular. This is definitely a site where results are going to vary widely. Do we recommend it? You bet.

- Buttocks. Liposuction will reduce your size—it can make you a teeny weeny size 4 or 6—but you may end up with a "flat ass." You might even get a saggy one. We hate to tell you, girlfriends, but the butt you dream about, the one you had when you were fifteen?—you still can have it, or almost, but you need a surgeon who can do a beautiful buttock tuck . . . and then you will have a scar.

- Upper inner thighs. This procedure is much requested, and very badly needed by most women, and almost guaranteed to leave you with loose skin. Even twenty-four-year-old girlfriend Julia was left with "unsightly" sagging. It's not age-related; it's site-related. Like your butt, this area will only give you the look you want if you're willing to have scars from a thighplasty.

- Back of your thighs, above the knee. Liposuction will give you a lovely contour—like you've been doing hamstring exercises for decades. But your skin tone and cellulite problem might make you less than perfect without your clothes on. This site is not one of liposuction's best bets. It will work, but there is a trade-off of dimpled skin (Lillis, 975).

- Knees. You know that fat you hate, the stuff that may be hanging over your knee? Say good-bye, because this area comes out great with liposuction.

- Calves and ankles. And you thought *you* were stuck with heavy legs for life! Somebody ought to tell Hillary Clinton about this one. (Are you mentally arguing that she probably doesn't care? Oh, come on! She has been dressing her whole life to "minimize" her thick calves and ankles. Take a look at her clothes choices). Your calves and ankles can slim down, with no loose skin; in fact, you can have fantastic results if a good plastic surgeon performs liposuction here for you. Please note, you should have *very strict* leg elevation for four to seven days post-op, and surgical-grade compression hose, but this is one of those sites where a radical change in appearance can make a difference in your everyday life (Ersek and Salisbury, 880–83). Barb Gresh had this surgery at the same time as her buttock tuck. She is thrilled.

- Upper arms. Controversy abounds about "bingo arms." You might get great results with excellent skin contraction, or you might have flab flapping in the breeze. It might be worth a try before opting for the long, visible scar of a "brachioplasty" (surgical reduction of the arms). One upscale magazine article recommended ultrasound liposuction for arms. It reports, "In ultrasonic liposuction, the fat is first emulsified, then sucked out. In the liquification process, heat is generated which almost 'shrink-wraps' the skin, leaving behind toned upper arms."

("Chat with Charlie," *Form and Figure,* Winter 1999, page 81).
We respectfully disagree! There is no evidence that ultrasound
improves skin retraction. Sorry, Charlie, but arms are a tough
place to get good results from any form of liposuction.

- Pubic fat pads. Oh Lord, are they the worst, or what? Girlfriends, you may have to alert your surgeon, but if you have a
fat Venus mound, it will look worse after a tummy tuck if you
don't have the fat sucked out. Think about your profile—flat
stomach and protruding pubic area. Not a pretty sight. You'll
get great liposuction results. Girlfriend Lisa asked me to be sure
to mention this. She went back in for a "touch-up" to have it
done. (Girlfriends, just a note to remember: A "touch-up" is
really a whole liposuction procedure. It may not be for a large
area, but it is a separate operation . . . and it entails all the usual
costs, though you might get a discount. Lisa has had a total of
twelve plastic surgery procedures—so far!)

- Fat over the coccyx bone. You know, where your spine meets
your butt. If you have fat removed from your waist and hips, be
sure this fat is sucked out too. The skin contracts well . . . and
your profile will be much nicer (Lillis, 976).

Going In to Go Under

Before you have any procedure, including liposuction, carefully go
over chapter 15: "Preparing Mentally and Physically for Surgery."
No matter what surgery you are scheduling, the steps in getting
ready are critically important.

Once the day arrives and you are ready for the procedure, the
doctor carefully draws on your skin where he or she is going to
remove the excess fat. Next, the doctor injects a large amount of
diluted local anesthetic solution into the area you are having "contoured." This numbs the area and reduces bleeding.

The truth about cuts and scars.

After the area to be treated is ready, a small incision (1/4 inch or smaller) is made in the skin, and a tube called a blunt-tipped cannula is inserted. These incisions are hidden as much as possible in the natural folds and creases of your body, in the pubic hair, navel, or buttock fold. But that isn't always possible, and you may have little scars where the incision is made. The scars are red or pigmented for six weeks; then they gradually pale out until they are almost imperceptible a year after surgery. However, there are no guarantees. Girlfriend Julie, who has extremely fair and fragile skin, still has some pink scars two years after her procedure. You need to be aware that all these scars are permanent, and their size and final appearance is not predictable.

Some of these incisions have no stitches at all. Most of the stitches that are used will dissolve; however, sometimes stitches have to be removed a week after surgery.

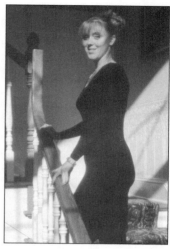

Here's Julie after liposuction. The camera adds ten pounds—she's super slim!

ULTRASOUND LIPOSUCTION (UAL)—IS IT BETTER?

The technique called ultrasound-assisted lipoplasty was developed over a decade ago in Torino, Italy, by Michele Zocchi. The media jumped on this technique and spread the word that it caused less bruising and bleeding, gave better results, and promoted faster healing. Unfortunately, none of that is proving true in controlled studies (Fodor and Watson, 1103). What studies did find were some added risks.

But wait! That doesn't mean ultrasound liposuction is bad.

UAL has its place, an important one. Here it is: The alternative form of liposuction, suction-assisted liposuction surgery, takes tremendous physical effort by the doctor. The sheer expenditure of energy, and the laborious, time-consuming nature of SAL once limited how much fat could be removed from a patient, even after surgeons found ways to make a large volume of fat removal safe. Then came UAL. UAL is much easier on the surgeon. It requires far less physical effort. It allows him or her to work faster. Which would you rather have working on you—an exhausted surgeon with aching arms, or one feeling strong throughout the surgery? UAL has become an invaluable tool in surgical fat reduction. If it is not quite the miracle we hoped for, UAL still deserves a prominent place in liposuction surgeries.

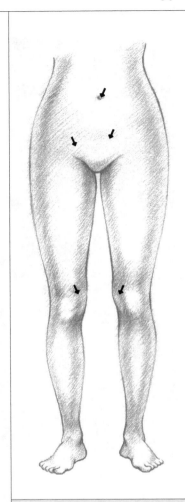

Liposuction incisions

The bottom line is that liposuction requires some cutting, and the more areas of the body you have done, the more places you will have little scars. It is one of the trade-offs. Expect it.

Out, out, damned fat!

Okay, there you are on the table, your mind in the twilight zone, and your legs perhaps spread in a frog-like position. It's a good thing you're unconscious; you are not looking your most attractive and your dignity is in the toilet. The area on your body to be suctioned has been flooded with a solution that contains an anesthetic such as Xylocaine, epinephrine, and other fluids (this is called the "tumescent" technique). The cut has been made. Now it's time to get out the fat.

The small, hollow cannula, which is attached to a vacuum source, is inserted into the fatty area. The fat is loosened from surrounding tissue by moving the tube back and forth Did we say something about moving? Oh yes, the tube "moves," with a great deal of effort. The surgeon looks as if he is using a Roto-Rooter on a clog that doesn't bulge. The fat does not go without a fight! It takes a lot of effort and pushing and pulling on the part of the doctor to get that fat loose.

Next the fat is sucked out though the tube, which is attached to a vacuum pump. Think about that the next time you're doing your rugs.

If you've never seen what your fat actually looks like, think chicken fat. Chicken fat is closer in color and texture to human fat than beef fat is. Human fat is lumpy, yellow, and definitely not a pretty sight. Since the fat that is removed from your body by liposuction is put in a container, measured, and photographed, you will get to see it firsthand.

Generally no more than four or five pounds of fat are removed at one time, though Sheri had nine pounds taken. Larger volume liposuction can even average ten to fifteen pounds. It depends on your overall height, weight, and state of health. If you have a great deal to be removed, you may need a second procedure, which the physician usually discounts in cost (for example, 80 percent of the first procedure's cost).

When the fat is sucked out, blood and body fluids come along with it. Although liposuction techniques have been improved to reduce blood loss, you can still lose a significant amount. For that reason, women who are having large amounts of fat removed may be asked to give blood ahead of time for a transfusion afterward. Although some doctors don't do this, studies are showing that women with *large* amounts of fat removed by liposuction, recover faster and feel stronger when they do have the transfusion of their own blood. Ask your doctor about doing this if you plan on having more than four or five pounds removed. You might also be given an iron supplement after surgery to help get your strength and blood count back.

How long will you be on the table? It depends on whether you are having liposuction alone or along with another procedure. The liposuction itself can last between one and three hours.

After the sucking.

Immediately after surgery, before you even get into the recovery room, you will be put into a special compression girdle, hereafter called "the garment"—Absolutely hideous-looking and crotchless, the garment looks so anti-sexy you might think of it as a birth-control device.

But the garment is your key to good results. Love it, even though you might hate the way it looks.

Susan explains the need for the garment like this:

Fat supports the skin. When the fat is removed, your skin has nothing to adhere to. It's loose. It hangs. The garment presses the skin against the muscle and whatever fat still remains. The garment holds the two surfaces together, and hopefully they will heal together, with the skin attached to a firm foundation, not flapping around or hanging. To get good results and good skin retraction you need [to wear] the garment continuously!

Some styles of the garment go from beneath your boobs to mid-thigh. They generally have two zippers, one on each side. They look like your grandmother's girdles. Some go all the way to your ankles. Some have suspenders. Most of them are white or flesh-colored, but they do come in black, with a little lace; this does not make them any more attractive. You will have the garment on day and night for one week after surgery. Then you will be wearing it during the day for a long time—at least a month. According to girl-friends we spoke to, they felt that the longer you can tolerate wearing the garment, the better the results. They also advocated wearing the garment if you are going to do anything strenuous for up to three months after surgery. Girlfriend Barbara S. felt that her wonderful, thorough healing and "nice" scar after her liposuction and tummy tuck was directly related to her wearing the garment when she felt fatigued from exertion. She believed, perhaps rightly, that she should avoid any strain on the abdomen.

If you have liposuction on your legs, you can, with your doctor's approval, replace the garment with high-quality tights after the first week. You need Lycra tights that really hug your legs, like the ones you always wanted to wear to aerobics class but never dared to until now. *Compression stockings for varicose veins will not work!* That type of stocking is tight on the lower leg but loosens up on the upper. You need steady, even tightness from ankle to hip.

The garments aren't cheap by any means, but you might want to get two if your doctor does not provide them. One, and often two, are included in the price of the procedure. The first garment put on you after surgery is probably going to get soiled from seepage (and from performing your normal bodily functions!). You don't want to keep it off even for a short time that first week, so make sure you do have two. Then you can at least launder one. For extended wear, an extra takes the pressure off having to wash it at night to put back on in the morning.

Here's a special note if you have liposuction to reduce your granny arms. This garment is especially difficult to tolerate because it is so tight and impedes movement. A girlfriend who is a beautician felt the garment greatly restricted her movement. Also, remember that loose skin on the arms will be worsened by liposuction. If you have bingo arms that truly flap, you will probably have to have a brachioplasty (see pages 88–89).

Your surgeon may give you post-operative instructions. Be sure to read them and follow them carefully. But sometimes you might not get instructions, so we have provided general guidelines in chapter 15. The information answers some of your questions and gives you a clear picture of what to expect after this surgery. However, follow your own surgeon's advice if there is a conflict. *Don't do anything on your own, and don't do anything simply because that's what a girlfriend did.*

Girlfriends' Advice for Before Surgery

- Buy Lycra tights to replace the dreaded garment when your doctor gives the okay.

- Have some loose, comfortable pants or sweats on hand to cover the garment, and to disguise your swelling.

- Have some new clothes waiting—a size or two smaller!

Girlfriends' Tips for Your Recovery

For most girlfriends, recovery from liposuction is a breeze. They are out hopping around in forty-eight hours. But there are some precautions to take, so following are girlfriends' tips to help protect your health, and to help you get the great results you want.

- Two to three days after the procedure most women can comfortably drive a car. You really can't go out until that first shower at any rate, because you're not going to smell very good. Until then, you are not going to want to be around anyone but very good friends and lovers . . . or your mother.

- After a week you can return to work if your job doesn't entail much physical activity. However, some tough girlfriends, like Barb Gresh, went back after four days.

- Take ten days to two weeks off if your job involves hard physical activity (lifting patients or carrying trays, for example).

- As soon as you feel well enough, begin leisurely walking for exercise. Take two weeks before you get back on an exercise bike. Wait three weeks until you go back to the gym for aerobics or weight training. Don't push it. You just paid a lot of money for this procedure; give yourself the maximum healing time possible.

- For a minimum of four to six months after surgery, wear a sunblock with SPF 15 or higher on all incisions and areas affected by your liposuction. The sun interferes with healing and may cause excessive redness and itching. It can also cause hyperpigmentation (darker skin).

What to Expect Medically After Liposuction

Done by a board-certified plastic surgeon, liposuction is extremely safe. After surgery it is normal to experience the following symptoms.

- A *small* amount of bloody drainage for twenty-four hours or so.

- Tiredness, fatigue, grogginess, or forgetfulness. You will probably feel "wiped out" the day after surgery, more from the anesthesia than anything else.

- Soreness. You may not want to move around very much for the first forty-eight hours.

- Bruising and swelling of the liposuction sites. Normally, bruising is completely resolved by three weeks.

- Swelling of the feet and ankles is common after liposuction. This is more of a nuisance than a medical problem. Don't be concerned if swelling occurs.

- Mild discomfort. You should *not* experience severe pain after this procedure. However, you might feel a brief, shooting pain. This can happen for several weeks after surgery. Not

BEWARE "THE SPONGE"

During the first week following surgery, the only time you will take off the garment is for your Reston sponge removal. Okay, what's *that*?

Reston foam sponges are applied to your body after surgery. The sponges help prevent bruising, protect the treated areas, and promote the development of smooth skin. On the third or fourth day after surgery, you will be instructed to remove the Reston foam sponges. Then you can shower.

Sometimes this removal is a breeze. The instructions you get from the doctor will probably tell you to apply mineral oil to lubricate the skin before removing the sponges. Then they are supposed to come off easily. But you might want to get help with the process.

The girlfriends who work in Susan's day spa, seeing the results of liposuction close at hand, began having the procedure themselves. They also began helping each other remove the Reston sponges. This became a regular routine whenever a friend or employee had liposuction. Soon, Susan began offering Reston sponge removal sessions to patients—and everybody loves it.

For some girlfriends, the sponges practically fall off. But sometimes the Reston sponges are more like having adhesive pulled off. Ouch! Most girlfriends felt mild discomfort, if anything. Teresa felt the slow pulling off of the sponges was a torment; she wanted them pulled off with one big yank. This is *not* a good idea.

everyone experiences this, but it is a normal occurrence for many women.

- Numbness. Nerves to the skin may be interrupted during surgery. This is more a nuisance than a medical problem and feeling returns over several months. Occasionally, some diminished sensitivity may last indefinitely in spots.

- Lumpy areas. Some of these can be smoothed out by self-massage or a professional massage during the healing phase. If they do not go away, try the subdermal therapy described on pages 65–66 after you are completely healed in six months.

- Redness around incision sites. This will fade in three to four months.

- Flaky, peeling surface skin. Anytime there is edema (swelling), you will find the top layer of skin sloughs off when the swelling goes down. This is harmless, and more a cosmetic nuisance than anything else.

- Scars. All scars tend to fade with time. However, the final width, height, color, and appearance cannot be predicted before surgery. The final outcome depends on a variety of factors including genetics, individual skin chemistry, nutrition, smoking, post-operative care, and one's overall capacity for healing.

You may not see an immediate reduction in weight because you are swollen. The same holds true for clothing size—although you should see a drop of from one to three clothing sizes (or more) once the swelling resolves. Expect to see gradual improvement in appearance for three to six months. As healing continues, the final result will emerge. *Do not judge your results before six months. Be patient.*

So how good are the results?

The results from liposuction can be dramatic. Girlfriend Barb Gresh went from a size 14 to a size 6, even a 4 with some clothes!

- If you develop pains in your chest or shortness of breath.
- If you develop pains in your lower legs.
- If there is excessive bleeding or swelling.
- If you develop an ulcer or an open wound.
- If you see any pus or red streaks at an incision site.

Your body can go from being totally out of proportion, to classically lovely. But don't expect perfection. *It is impossible to create the perfect body with liposuction.* We can't stress this strongly enough. You may get a vastly improved body, but it is not going to be perfect. And no matter how good the surgeon is, you may get uneven results and some other disadvantages of liposuction. However, you can have a second procedure at a later date to eliminate asymmetry—usually at a 20 percent discount—but it still costs!

Other shortcomings of liposuction.

There is a downside to liposuction. So let's get something straight immediately. If you think your legs are going to look great in a bathing suit after liposuction when they didn't before, think again.

Liposuction will improve your shape. It will reduce your volume. It will not get rid of bumps, lumps, dimpled skin, or loose skin. In fact, one of the side effects of liposuction is some lumpy areas. Chances are, if you had dimpled fat or cellulite before the procedure, it will be the same, or worse, afterward. *Liposuction is not a cure. In fact, it can intensify one thing you really hate: cellulite.*

The other major consequence of liposuction may be sagging or wrinkled skin. Ideally, after liposuction the skin retracts inward. The neck, calves, and ankles, for example, generally come out beautifully. But there is no way to predict how well your skin will

---

THE PURPLE SNAPPER

No one ever hinted such a thing could happen. But there you are. You just had liposuction and/or a tummy tuck and your pubic area—including your most private parts—look as if they were dipped in grape juice. Unbelievable. Totally gross. And because the garment is crotchless, there is your vibrantly colored crotch hanging out in the breeze. This is the "purple snapper" syndrome, one of those shocking conditions no one ever talks about. It will go away eventually—after it turns psychedelic colors of raspberry-red and urine-yellow. So rest assured, girlfriend, the "purple snapper" is perfectly natural.

contract. Age is not a factor, but age will influence healing time and the time before you see the final results (Goddio, 68). Genetics and the area of the body treated are the determinants of how you will look. Don't be surprised or disappointed if your thighs, abdomen, or butt sag (Goddio, 68). The only thing you can do is have a skin reduction to get rid of the excess.

Another relatively common complication is pigmentation, or dark areas, on the skin. No one is sure why this "staining" occurs, but it happens most frequently to girlfriends with olive or darker complexions. Most of the time the stains fade over a period of several months, but in some cases the staining may persist for up to and well over one year (Ersek and Burry, 380).

What about more serious complications? The really serious potential complication is an embolism, either fat or a blood clot—and death. This is most likely to happen when a patient has an underlying health problem, such as chronic high blood pressure or a heart problem, when too much of the "tumescent" solution is used, and when too much fat is extracted during one procedure. In the hands of a qualified, competent, board-certified plastic surgeon—the one you are going to pick—*this complication is rare.* Those "deaths on the table" during liposuction happen most often when the practitioner isn't qualified. So don't be lured into an unknown doctor's office by aggressive marketing that feeds into fantasy instead of reality. Don't be swayed by persuasive newspaper ads. The "surgeon" may not be a surgeon at all. The consequences of a hasty, "blind" choice can be fatal. (Schulte and Bergal, 1, 10A).

The need to maintain your reduction.

So you had liposuction. You can get into those slim jeans or a straight skirt. You look great—right now. But if you gain weight after you get liposuction, be ready to cry yourself a river. The fat can still go where it was sucked out if any fat cells are left there. But more likely it goes everywhere else, and *not* evenly. Your fat distribution works like those choices some mail-order houses give you: "If your first choice isn't available, please list your second." Well, your body sends the fat to your genetically preferred spots first. Once that now-limited seating is filled, the fat gets zipped over to second-choice spots: your neck, your shoulders, your back, behind your knees, and other places you never got fat before. Some girlfriends who continued their poor eating habits ended up looking like football players, with humongous *upper* bodies. Susan got little fat pockets right behind her knees (and Susan has a very low percentage of body fat).

What can you do? In your heart, you already know the answer. Exercise, and watch your calorie intake. You need a regular aerobic program to maintain the results of your liposuction. One doctor recommends a very gentle program: walking on a slightly inclined treadmill at a very slow rate—less than 3 miles per hour, 30 minutes a day, three to five days a week (Vash, 220). Girlfriend, anyone can do that!

However, vigorous sports and high-impact aerobics are prohibited for two to three weeks after surgery.

Now it's up to you.

Liposuction gives the most satisfactory results when it's used to correct a body that is grossly out of proportion. It is not recommended as a primary means of weight reduction. But for some very overweight women, it can be a significant way to improve body image and self-esteem. However, it should be part of a total program of weight reduction, diet, and exercise.

Think about the risks carefully before you decide—and have realistic expectations about the results. If you opt to do it with that mind-set, you will probably recuperate easily and love your look. There is a definite mind-body connection.

If you have any reservations, doubts, or fears, don't rush into anything. Take your time. Surgery is forever, and it's a big decision.

DON'T DIET BEFORE SURGERY

If you are planning liposuction surgery, it's no time to start dieting. You want to be strong and healthy when you have surgery. Dieting can cause imbalances in your body; it definitely stresses your system. After surgery, make significant changes in your diet. You just paid a great deal of money to look better. If you have to, tack your bill on your refrigerator door . . . and change your eating habits for the better.

Meanwhile, take out a gym membership and actually go. See what changes you can make in your body with weight training. Then you will know for sure which bulges will budge and which ones need to be sucked down the tube!

CELLULITE—IS THERE HELP? IS THERE HOPE?

Women have been complaining about cellulite for years. No doctors listened. They even told us it didn't exist. It was just fat, they said. Now, cellulite is getting some serious attention and some scientific investigation. So far there is no "cure." But at least the scientific community has decided it does exist, it is a problem worthy of study, and they may even have discovered what it is.

Here's the scoop from one scholarly article: Cellulite is caused when the fat (adipose tissue) extends up into the dermis because the connective tissue isn't strong enough to keep it from penetrating upward; the reason the connective tissue is weaker may be connected to the presence of androgens (a hormone). The areas where cellulite occurs are highly variable, but often happen in positions that tend to compress the adipose tissue in a specific area, enhancing the dimpling effect (in other words, when you sit on a chair your thighs look really bad) (Rosenbaum et al, 1934–39).

Guess what? Those topical cellulite creams don't work (Epstein et al, 304). The active ingredient in most of them is aminophylline. Manufacturers claim this substance inactivates the androgen receptors of the fat cells. Supposedly this helps activate "lipolysis"—or fat-burning. Sounds convincing, but that just doesn't happen. Fortunately, the aminophylline doesn't seem to get into your bloodstream to do any harm. On the downside, some of the other ingredients can cause the user to break out in a rash. Overall, the greatest harm is done to your pocketbook.

If studies can further pinpoint how to get the androgen back in balance and strengthen the connecting tissue, there may be a real "cure" for cellulite someday. In the meantime, weight loss and exercise will definitely minimize the amount of cellulite you have. And you may get some benefit from a very pleasant experience—massage (Epstein et al). Massage evidently can displace or destroy the "adipocytes." And massage is so beneficial to your health—particularly because it stimulates circulation and vastly decreases your stress level—we feel you should go for it, girl!

The Mystery of Mechanical Massage— Subdermal Therapy

Since massage *may* help reduce the appearance of cellulite, can deeper massage do a better job? It looks like the answer is yes. The technique is called "subdermal therapy," but you will see various brand names. The machine that administers the treatment combines massage with suction more powerful than an Electrolux™ vacuum cleaner. The machine, which is run over your body by a technician, pulls up and pummels the skin. It is supposed to squish the fat cells and iron them out.

Generally, a series of treatments (one manufacturer recommends fifteen) are needed in order to see any results. You start off with two sessions per week until your series is completed, then one session a month for maintenance. The program is combined with health and diet advice; particularly, to drink eight glasses of water a day. We applaud that. Your skin will love you . . . and maybe it will help your cellulite.

As far as subdermal therapy goes, we give it a cautious green light. The FDA has said subdermal therapy can officially claim to be a means of reducing the appearance of cellulite. If that sounds a bit lukewarm, it is still significant that the FDA has given it any legitimacy; there had to be measurable results for the therapy to get it.

Early reports are encouraging. Susan swore she saw some changes after just one session, but it is supposed to take three.

Another girlfriend's husband gave her the thumbs-up after he saw the results of three treatments. Another girlfriend we know lost a total of *eight inches* from her hips, thighs, and torso. Charlee tried it along with a weight-loss program. She definitely lost inches, but there is no way to determine if the subdermal therapy accelerated the results of the diet. She felt the experience was uncomfortable. Boy, did it pinch!

We think subdermal therapy is worth trying. At $75 on the average for a session, it is affordable—especially if you begin to see visible results after three sessions.

If subdermal therapy really does swoosh out cellulite, we propose giving the inventor a Nobel Prize.

3

Getting Out the Big Guns: The Tummy Tuck

Girlfriends, a tummy tuck (abdominoplasty) is major surgery, but it can be life-changing. It is a procedure you need to know about, even if you are lucky enough to never need it. Why? Because you do know someone—a friend, sister, cousin, or mother—who does.

The reasons for getting a tummy tuck can vary from desire for a totally flat stomach to wanting an abdominal area that will cause heartbreak beyond words. A tummy tuck can make a slightly flawed figure look like dynamite, or a tummy tuck can release a woman from the prison her body has become. If this last description does not fit you, think about someone close to you: a girlfriend who will never let anyone see her without clothes, who has not been to the beach for years, who can never put on a pair of jeans, or who can dream of sex, but it is only a dream, because she does not feel a man can ever want someone who looks like her.

Let's take a closer look at this surgery—the conditions it can help, what the procedure entails (including your new belly button), how quickly you will recover, what the trade-offs are, and what risks you need to consider.

Jelly Belly . . . and Other Reasons to Get Tucked

In 1998, 42,249 women had abdominoplasties according the American Society for Aesthetic Surgery. What prompted that many women to elect to undergo a serious operation?

One reason is a protruding abdomen. Any protruding abdomen is the result of weak or stretched abdominal muscles. Susan says to think of the elastic on your underwear: Once it loses its elasticity, it stays stretched. That pretty much describes your abdominal muscles. Forget crunches, leg lifts, and other forms of torture. Stretched muscles don't respond well to exercise; they just won't tighten up again. Thanks to your genes, you might have a fat pad right on top of these stretched or separated muscles. Dieting doesn't seem to reduce this annoying paunch, but any weight gain expands it with ease. Weak abdominal muscles are a cause of back pain—another factor for considering abdominoplasty (Toranto, 545).

Another reason for a tummy tuck is loose or flaccid skin. This can happen after pregnancy or weight loss. Charlee had a tummy tuck because of loose skin. She had experienced a quick weight gain, putting on thirty pounds one emotionally terrible year; then she got her head together and had a dramatic weight loss in six months. *Great,* she thought, *I'm back to my fighting weight of 120.* Not great—her stomach looked like a deflated balloon. If she leaned over, or knelt on her hands and knees, it just fell forward like a curtain of empty, loose skin. She couldn't believe it. She thought that in time and with enough trips to the gym it would shrink up again. Well, it didn't. Flaccid skin never does. Think of those Slim-Fast ads. Now think again, and figure out why you don't see the girls who lost sixty or seventy pounds posing in bathing suits. The fat may be gone, but the skin stays: wrinkled, elephant-like, droopy folds of skin. The diet gurus never warn us about this! Oh no, they just preach about getting the pounds off, and you'll be happy. You'll be happy if you're blessed with super skin retraction. Otherwise, girl-friends, you'll be in shock!

A third reason for a tummy tuck is stubborn obesity. Surgery is not a good way to lose weight. But for girlfriends like September (see pages 46–47), it is the only way. For them, it dramatically helped to improve body image and "jump-start" a life of healthier eating and exercise.

There is another reason for a tummy tuck, a problem that is still hidden behind closed doors. Even in these liberated days, when condoms and tampons are advertised on TV and nothing seems taboo on *Jerry Springer*, this problem is still . . .

The dirtiest little secret of pregnancy.

Short, upbeat, cute as can be, Barbara S. is wearing jeans and a sweater. What's so unusual about that? Well, for nearly twenty years Barbara couldn't wear any clothes except an oversized shirt that reached to midthighs over baggy pants or an elastic-waist skirt. She couldn't wear a dress. She couldn't put on a belt. She could never tuck in a blouse. Every piece of clothing she owned was designed to hide and accommodate an "apron" of skin that hung down from her abdomen to below her crotch. Even the girdle she wore continuously could not completely support it. What happened to Barbara is called "post-pregnancy syndrome," and it has devastated the lives of uncounted legions of women. Tragically, few of them ever talk about it.

Postpregnancy syndrome is characterized by distended skin with stretch marks, a relaxed abdomen, and a separation and stretching of the abdominal muscles (Muhlbauer). Sometimes, the inner thighs as well as the abdominal region are covered with folds of hanging flesh. It can even affect women in their twenties or thirties—after *one* pregnancy.

Words alone cannot convey the disfigurement of "postpreg-nancy syndrome"—or the guilt, shame, and self-blame women feel. They don't have that hanging flesh because they aren't going to the gym; they don't have it because they are fat, lazy, or sloppy. They need to understand they did nothing wrong to cause it. And women, no matter what their age or how long they have had the condition, need to know they don't have to suffer any longer. There is help. They can look completely normal again.

As Barbara explains,

This happened to me after I had my very first child. I wasn't Twiggy, but I certainly wasn't obese. I'm only five feet tall, and I gained a lot of weight during the pregnancy, over sixty pounds. After my daughter's birth, I was left with wide stretch marks across my entire middle, and my abdomen looked like a beach ball that lost its air. The skin hung straight down, covering my entire crotch area. My husband came home from Vietnam with an alcohol problem. When he saw me, the verbal abuse started and continued until I got up the nerve to walk out on him a decade later. He called me a "fat turkey fool" and other cruel words that shattered my self-esteem. He made a nasty comment about any food I ate. I became a secret eater, sneaking into the kitchen after everyone was asleep or had left for the day. I felt awful about myself, and my "apron" just got worse after I had my second daughter.

It not only looked terrible, it caused all sorts of health problems. It became chapped and raw underneath. My skin was stained and discolored. The hanging flesh caused hygiene problems. The weight of it pulling down caused excruciating back pain. It was a real disability. [Barbara was lucky because flesh rubbing against flesh can cause terrible ulcers, rashes, fistulas, circulation problems, and hinder movement (Matory et al, 976–77), which is why insurance should, and sometimes does, cover the correction of this problem!]

I never let my shape stop me. I started my own housecleaning business. I was a real dynamo, never stopping. But there were times my back pain was terrible. And I always looked fat.

My two girls were great. They never made me feel ashamed of how I looked. "You have to meet my mom," they always said as they introduced a schoolmate or a date. But after I had the tummy tuck, I put on a pair of slacks and a sweater to see the doctor for a checkup. My oldest daughter went along, and she said to the doctor, "This is the first time I've ever seen my mother look normal. I can see her hips." I was taken aback, because I never thought it bothered them.

All those years, it never occurred to me to have surgery. But I cleaned for a doctor, and one day he said to me, just in conversation, "You know, you can fix your stomach. You'll get around better. And it will probably stop your backache." I was so insulted! I thought, *Why, I zoom around! What does he mean, I'll get around better?* Then I began thinking about it. I found out my insurance would cover the cost. But I postponed the surgery for a whole year while I made up my mind I really wanted to do it.

The first thirty-six hours were tough after the surgery. There was a lot of pain right in the beginning, and a burning feeling. But once the drain was out, I healed very quickly. I didn't like being confined. Within seven days I was up and about. And the doctor was right. I didn't realize what a burden I had been lugging around all those years. Now, I fly when I work. My back pain is gone. But something else is gone, too, a pain inside me that I never talked about.

And I'll tell you something else. My ex-husband passed away as a result of his alcoholism. At the end, he was

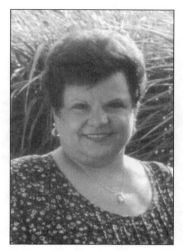

Barbara S., mother of two grown daughters, is ready to take on the world.

grossly obese. They even had to order a special casket to fit him in. I never saw or spoke to him in the years after our divorce, but my daughters asked me to go to the funeral. I put on a straight *knit* skirt and high heels. I looked terrific. I sailed into the funeral home and didn't even acknowledge the stares of his family, who never liked me. I knew I looked great. I went up to the casket and looked at that abusive SOB. I didn't feel bad for him at all. "Who is the fat turkey fool bastard now?" I said, and a smile started from my toes and went all the way to the top of my head. I was grinning, I tell you. Then I turned around, held my head high, and strode out.

Preparing for the surgery.

Review chapter 15 on getting ready for surgery, and follow all of your doctor's instructions to the letter.

NAUGHTY NANETTE AND THE CLOSE SHAVE

Girlfriends, the tummy tuck is one of those operations where you have to shave the pubic area before surgery. Now, listen carefully, because we are going to get down and dirty here, and shockingly honest. A common reaction among girlfriends after this shave is to continue to keep the pubic area clean-shaven . . . permanently.

Why? First of all, many men find a shaved "pussy" very erotic. Some husbands, seeing not only a wife's newly flat and toned stomach, but also her clean-as-a-whistle snatch, express a preference for the look, perhaps daring to say so for the first time. A large number of tummy-tuck veterans have continued shaving to please their men.

There is another deeper, darker reason—so, menopausal girlfriends, lend us your ears. As you age, your pubic hair gets sparse. It turns gray or white. It looks straggly and extremely unattractive. What can a woman do? She may have the face and body of a thirty-year-old, and the bush of an old lady. Women can't safely dye the hair in this area, and so far as we know, there are no pubic-hair transplants. So shave. Be daring. Be risqué. Be erotic. Be smart enough to get rid of the whole, hormonally caused problem. But girlfriends, this shaving is a secret. Nobody but your lover will ever know unless you tell them . . . and oh, how deliciously naughty!

Make arrangements to be out of work for a week, but also create a contingency plan to handle work and home responsibilities if you must convalesce longer. Consider putting together a "team" to help handle your normal tasks and responsibilities. This may depend on how open you are being about your surgery, but since women sometimes have abdominal surgery for gynecological reasons, a convincing cover story should be easy.

On the table.

A full abdominoplasty may be performed under general anesthesia, which means you are asleep and receiving help breathing throughout the entire procedure. However, this operation is being performed more frequently under local anesthesia and intravenous sedation, depending on your individual case and the doctor's evaluation. Many tummy tucks are done on an outpatient basis, meaning you go home soon after the surgery is performed. If insurance is covering the procedure, or if the surgeon decides it is appropriate for you, a hospital stay of two or three days may be required. But more and more, many tucks are being performed safely in an office facility. Tummy tucks are often combined with liposuction, tubal ligation, hysterectomy, breast enlargement, breast reduction, gallbladder surgery, or even face-lifts.

Although there are several adominoplasty procedures from which to choose, the one most frequently used by physicians involves a ∪-shaped incision made below one hip bone and across the pubic area to under the other hip bone. The doctor may ask you to wear your bathing suit of choice so he can place the incision where it won't show. A second incision is made around the navel.

Next, the surgeon separates the skin from the abdominal wall and lifts it up to the breastbone. Once that is done, he will suture loose or stretched out muscles in your abdomen to stop them from sagging. The fat that has made that annoying belly bulge is removed, and the skin is lowered back over the abdomen, put in place, and the excess skin is cut away, creating a beautiful, flat, tight stomach.

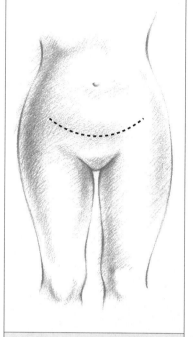

Abdominoplasty incision

But, before the incisions are closed with small sutures, your belly button is reconstructed.

Next, one or more drains are inserted near the sutures to eliminate fluid buildup. Drains are long latex tubes with holes in them. The end will protrude from your incision and drip a bloody- to pinkish-colored watery discharge.

You may also have a urinary catheter in place for one to two days after surgery. Girlfriends, everyone *hates* the idea of a catheter before surgery. Everyone loves having one in after surgery. It is inserted while you are asleep, so you won't feel it. It doesn't hurt to have it removed. And you will bless it during the first twenty-four hours after surgery because you will not have to move to pee.

You will definitely be put into a compression garment (see all the details on the garment in chapter 2 on liposuction). It helps reduce swelling and gives support to your belly. It makes for a faster, smoother recovery period.

You will need someone to drive you home after surgery.

BUTTON, BUTTON, WHO'S GOT THE BELLY BUTTON?

The umbilicus is the only normal scar on the body, the absence of which may be distressing" (Baroudi). If you opt for a tummy tuck, be prepared for the fact that you are about to get a new navel. For some women, whose navels have been stretched out of shape or herniated by childbirth, this is welcome news. For others, this revision is a shock. Whether you're an innie or an outie, you are more attached to this "normal scar" than you may think. Discuss your new belly button with your surgeon before the operation. If you have strong preferences about size or shape, let your doctor know. You might want to see other belly buttons he or she has reconstructed. Some women complain that their new belly button is too small. The medical literature reports the case of a fifty-one-year-old woman with "stenosis" (a narrowing) of her new navel. She complained that her boyfriend was not able to sip champagne from it (Baack, et al, 231). And expect to have stitches in your navel after the surgery. The scar, however, should be hidden inside where it can't be noticed.

Girlfriends' Tips for Recovering Safely

Follow your surgeon's instructions to the letter. There will be pain for the first two days after abdominoplasty, and you will be given pain medication. Usually by day three or four, no pain medication is needed. Also, since you have a sizable incision, you may be applying a topical ointment. You will walk slightly hunched over for two to three days after surgery to avoid putting any tension on the incision. You will gradually be able to straighten up as your skin adjusts to your new body contour.

If you must cough, sneeze, or laugh during the first few days after the procedure, hold a pillow over your belly to relieve the pressure on the muscles. Do the same thing when you have a bowel movement.

You won't be able to shower until the drain is removed. Do not even think about taking a bath; you'd contaminate the incisions.

When you get the okay to shower, be sure you have help. You will likely be lightheaded, and fainting is a real possibility. *Do not try to shower when you are alone!*

A small amount of bloody drainage on the bandages is expected for three to five days after the surgery. You can expect some discomfort, but this should be readily relieved by the pain medication.

Recovery Time for a Tummy Tuck

Most girlfriends can return to work a week after a full tummy tuck, or four to five days after a mini-tuck. But this can vary. Plan on a week, but leave yourself some wriggle room if you want more time. September breezed back to her job in sales in five days. Sheri also returned to work quickly, but with her strenuous job as a surgical nurse, she pushed herself too much and got an infection at the incision site. With a tummy tuck, please take your time before resuming normal activities. It is okay to pamper yourself.

WHEN TO CALL YOUR DOCTOR

If your belly becomes noticeably larger and this enlargement is associated with more pain, bruising, and tightness, call your doctor immediately.

Arrange for help with children and housework during your recovery period.

Strenuous sporting activities, or any other activity that will increase your heart rate or blood pressure, is strictly forbidden for at least two weeks after an abdominoplasty or until your doctor gives you the okay.

That was the formal, official description. Here is the real deal.

You will remember little to nothing of the operation before waking up in the recovery room where you will still be totally out of it. One awareness will penetrate the fog clouding your brain: Something major has happened to your body. You know that you have been wounded. If this were a Western, you would feel like the guy who lost the draw and has been shot in the gut—and you are hoping to be shot again to be put out of your misery. You will not be perky and cheery and ready to roll. If you are in a hospital, you will want only to go back to sleep or get an ice sliver to suck on because your mouth feels like the Sahara. You will not want visitors, conversation, or anything but your pain medication.

If the procedure is performed on an outpatient basis, not only do you need "someone" to drive you home, *you need someone*

PET ALERT

You love your cat or dog so much you let him sleep on the bed. A pet offers comfort when you're not feeling well. *But not this time.* You need to keep your distance from your pets until your incision is healed after an abdominoplasty or any other major surgery. We had one girlfriend, a nurse, who kept getting stubborn infections after her surgery. Nobody could figure out why until a laboratory culture identified the source of her infection—cat-scratch fever. You can't risk the chance of infection, and cat dander, flea dirt, hair, or other contaminants don't belong where there is an open wound (including your face after skin resurfacing!). If you do stroke your cat or dog, keep antibacterial wipes, or an antibacterial lotion, handy. And keep pets off the bed or couch where you are convalescing. No cheating! No exceptions!

strong enough to hold you up, get you into the car, get you out of the car, and keep you from doing a nosedive onto the driveway. Arrange to be escorted by two girlfriends, or a burly guy . . . though it better be a guy you know well, especially if you start heaving or passing out.

When you get home you will be in a daze for the next twenty four hours. If you have a catheter in place you won't have to get up to pee. But if you don't have one, use a bedpan. Have one handy. *Don't* try to get up. *Don't* attempt to climb stairs. If your bedroom is on the second floor, set up the sofa or a daybed in the living room. Pray you won't need to have a bowel movement; take the pillow along to press against your abdomen while you curse, yell, or cry.

Sex? Don't even think about it. In fact, you *won't* even think about it. Even after the first two weeks, if the lover in your life asks if you are ready for it, your answer will be: "Touch me, and you're a dead man."

Will you really walk hunched over? Chances are, there is no way humanly possible that you will be able to straighten up. You will wish you could walk with your head at crotch level. You'll move slowly . . . very slowly. At first, you probably won't be able to sit up without help. You won't want to turn over or move. You will want to lie there on your back, totally motionless, and pray for unconsciousness.

If you are sick from the anesthesia and feel nauseous, throwing up will be an experience. Try to skip that bit of torture by immediately calling your doctor and getting a suppository. (Some doctors now routinely have a suppository inserted before you wake up from the surgery, and it has eliminated much of this suffering.)

Suffering? You bet. Don't plan on seeing anyone other than the person who is waiting on you hand and foot. Hopefully, it will be your mother. No one else will want to put up with you. If your mother—or a compassionate, patient, and sensitive significant other—is not available (this eliminates a majority of men), you might want to hire a professional for a day or two. Then you can be as ungracious as you want to be without hurting anyone's feelings. And if you pee, bleed, or throw up on something you shouldn't, they're not going to go ballistic.

If you don't have anyone you can count on—if you have young children who will scream and cry when they see you and fling their bodies against your stomach . . . if you are the pillar who supports your house, and everyone else is helpless—*ask to stay in the hospital.* It will be a nightmare if you don't. You need to be taken care of for a few days. This is serious surgery. If you've already had a face-lift, *that* was a walk in the park. A tummy tuck is a marathon run.

Individual experiences vary. You may breeze through it. You may just snooze for a few days and watch old movies on TV. But be advised that you might have a rough forty-eight hours—and girl-friend, *do* call the doctor if you have a rough time of it. First, you need to make sure nothing is going wrong. Second, you can get medication to help make things easier.

After the first two days you will start feeling better quickly. You will feel like showing off your belly even with stitches and bruising. It will look incredibly good. You will be dreaming of halter tops and bikinis, or loose-waisted jeans dipping down to show your belly button. Think of those sexy, slim ingénues adorning the cover of *Rolling Stone* magazine. Oh yes, your tummy looks fantas-tic. But take it slow. Put a chair in the shower every time you take one. Don't make the water too hot. You might not be able to step over the edge of the tub without help. Again, this is not a surgery where you want to tough it out alone. Put your safety, health, and comfort before your pride and independence.

Don't think about doing aerobics for a good three weeks—and even that is ridiculously optimistic. Start thinking in terms of months. If you weight-train, take it easy. If you feel any strain on your abdomen, stop. You want your incision to heal into a nice, thin little line. Don't stretch it! If you are a golfer, see how it feels when you swing. You should be fine after three weeks. Skiing, tennis, or other high-impact, high-movement sports should be deferred as long as possible. Use your common sense.

COMPLICATIONS

One of the most common complications is infection, affecting about 1 percent of patients (Hester, 1000). Sheri developed an infection at the incision site. Charlee had a mild one at the navel. Anne got her navel pierced a few weeks afterward, got a reaction to the "ring," and wished she never dreamed up the whole wild idea. The abdomen is an area easily contaminated. Be vigilant, and if you develop redness, pus, or swelling at an incision site, tell your doctor immediately. The earlier you treat it, the faster you'll heal.

Other complications are seroma (fluid under the skin that can be easily aspirated out), or a minor skin slough, or loss of skin that causes an opening at the incision site. (Loss of skin happens most frequently to smokers!) The opening will heal in time, and your doctor will help you resolve the problem. It may not even make your scarring worse.

If you sunbathe, it can make your scar darker through hyperpigmentation. Don't expose your body to the sun. Use a self-tanner. If your scar is dark even without the sun, you can start a regimen of Retin-A® and bleaching cream. Ask your doctor about it.

The most serious complication of a tummy tuck is a blood clot or embolism. With a competent surgeon, your risk is very small. *Some of the symptoms of an embolism are pain and swelling in the lower legs, pain in the chest, or shortness of breath. This is a very serious condition. Do not hesitate to get medical help immediately.*

The best way to safeguard yourself against complications like these is, first, to feel confident in your doctor. Then, be sure you fully disclosure to him or her your health problems—if you are taking oral contraceptives or hormone-replacement therapy, if you take laxatives on a regular basis, or if you have an eating disorder, such as bulimia. *Do not keep any secrets from your surgeon; your life may depend on it.* Research now shows that age itself is not a risk factor; rather, general health is. And a definite risk factor is obesity (Hester, 999).

The trade-off.

The downside of a tummy tuck is a scar. This scar is easily hidden and usually follows your bikini line. Even if it extends around your hip area, you can cover it with your bathing suit or undies. In most cases the scar fades to a pencil-thin white line. Occasionally, parts will stay pinkish or purplish, and you might get "dog-ears" where it meets your hips, especially if you gain weight after the procedure. These are minor imperfections, and your surgeon will "correct" them. Remember, however, you may have to pay for the corrections, although dog-ears may be fixed for free.

Every girlfriend we know who has had a tummy tuck is thrilled with the results. All of them say it was worth it, even if they had some complications during the recovery period. The benefits are dramatic—the surgery often changes not only body image, but lives.

AND ONE MORE THING GIRLFRIENDS ASK ABOUT . . . PREGNANCY AFTER ABDOMINOPLASTY

Most girlfriends wait until after they have their children before having a tummy tuck. But accidents do happen, and so do circumstances in life and love. You can get pregnant after a tummy tuck. However, you need to alert your ob/gyn who might wish to consult with your plastic surgeon. The pregnancy may need to be monitored more closely than usual. A very conservative surgeon might advise against pregnancy, but certainly get a second opinion if you get pregnant and are advised to terminate it. This should not be necessary (Menz, 378).

THE BOTTOM LINE

It is essential to go into surgery feeling confident and sure that you want to do it. While feeling a little nervous and anxious is normal, any deep-seated fears or feelings of uncertainty mean you should not proceed with the surgery. Listen to your body. Listen to your heart. Listen to your doctor. *Don't listen to your friends or relatives.* The decision whether or not to have surgery is between you and your surgeon. It should not be made by anyone else, even a loved one. *Do what is right for you.*

4

OTHER NIPS AND TUCKS

Liposuction will suck out your fat. A tummy tuck will firm up your abdomen. But girlfriends, when the fat is gone, when the years go by, and when gravity tugs, we are left with another problem: loose, flabby, dimpled, hanging skin. There is help, but also a trade-off: scars. Right now, girlfriends, no one knows how to shrink skin or put the snap back in the elastic. The only way to fix the problem is to cut off the excess.

For many girlfriends, a scar is no biggie. What is intolerable is looking like an empty sack or "wearing" skin that makes you look 102 years old when you are thirty-five. As September confessed, after several surgeries, right now her body without clothes looks like a road map, but in clothes she looks great. She feels positive about her body image. Scars fade, or are easily hidden. But thighs dimpled with cellulite, and fat hanging over your knees will keep you from wearing shorts, a shorter skirt, and, of course, a bathing suit. How much longer are you going to sit out the summer in slacks?

THE PINCH TEST

How much extra skin do you have? If it's not immediately obvious, do the pinch test. (This is what the surgeon does when he marks your skin before surgery.) Here's how to do it: Take your thumb and index finger and gingerly squeeze redundant (loose) skin together. Take a marker and make dots along the top of the fold and along the bottom. Let go. Connect the dots and you can see the amount of skin that needs to be removed.

You can also do this pinch test without a pen. For example, just grab the excess skin and fat over your hips and gently pull up until the wrinkles and dimples on the side of your buttocks and legs disappear. Do the same for the top of your legs. Try it under your bra line, for your waist. Then try it with the flab sticking out between your bra and your armpit. Pinch any of the places where your excess skin (and the fat underneath it) is making you miserable about your looks. Any of this excess can be taken off with skin-reduction techniques, sometimes combined with liposuction.

THE WEIGHT-REDUCTION HOAX

Maybe you've been fat since childhood and have suffered silently with all the taunts and rejection that come with being overweight in our society. Maybe you gained weight during pregnancy and didn't lose it after your child was born. Maybe you just steadily added a pound or two over the years and ended up looking like your mother! Finally, after many tries and much deprivation, you took the weight off. You lost one hundred pounds, or sixty, or maybe just thirty. Instead of having the figure you dreamed about, you are depressed every time you look in the mirror.

The truth is, significant weight loss leaves you hanging! You've lost the weight, but your loose flesh looks so bad you wonder why you went through the struggle. Maybe you have even started eating again because you still hate the way you look. You need to know that your body can look as lovely as you fantasized it would be.

Be aware that you may need more than one procedure. You need to talk over the stages of skin reduction with your doctor. To give you an idea of what can be done, we've listed the most common types of operations. All of them can be done with local anesthetic and intravenous sedation in a fully equipped office operating facility:

- The Belt Abdominoplasty, or an abdominoplasty with a hip-plasty, is a tummy tuck where the incision continues around your hips to partly or completely encircle your trunk. The recovery does not differ from that of a regular tummy tuck. The benefit—firm, tight skin from back to front, from the hips down. The trade-off—a long scar, which can usually be hidden by a bathing suit bottom or your underpants.

- The buttock tuck fixes your backside, and it is often combined with liposuction. "Make my backside look like a

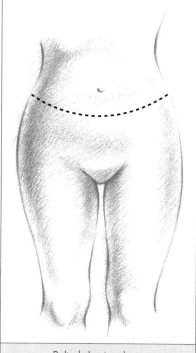

Belt abdominoplasty

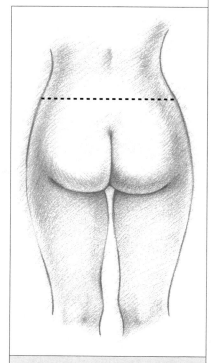

Belt abdominoplasty

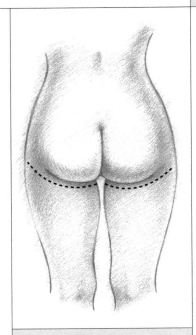

Buttock Tuck

fifteen-year-old's," Barb Gresh pleaded. Susan warned her it would look good, but probably not quite like a high-school kid's. Well, seeing is believing. There's a scar on the bottom of both her cheeks, but Barbara's got the cutest, perkiest, smoothest little behind you can imagine. It certainly could belong to a teenager.

How bad is a buttock tuck? None of the girlfriends we spoke to complained. They quickly glossed over some discomfort during the first day or two—and the inconvenience of not being able to sit! Teresa had a butt tuck with liposuction on her lateral thighs. "One of my legs was a full one inch bigger than the other. I couldn't wear leggings without feeling self-conscious," she explained. She felt so good after her procedure that she cooked a Thanksgiving Dinner for fourteen a week after her surgery.

Our girlfriends also had some great tips for coping with the inability to bend over. From Teresa:

The post-op instructions called for a few days of bed rest and for a week of keeping your knees bent and feet elevated while lying down. Pillows are awkward and hard to keep in position. What worked great under my knees was one of those wedge-shaped reading pillows with armrests. I had one covered with silky material, not corduroy, so I was able to easily reposition it by pulling on the arms, which were turned toward me. It worked beautifully.

Also, the instructions said to drink lots of Gatorade after the operation. I woke up starved, by the way, and the nurses had a bagel waiting for me in the recovery room! I had no nausea or ill-effects from the anesthesia. I felt great. I had Gatorade in a cooler in the car so I could continue to drink all the way home. I really forced fluids for three days, and I think it helped me heal better.

Speaking of drinking a great deal—what goes in, must come out. And after a buttock tuck, you can't sit down. The standard way to pee standing up is to use a cup. This can be messy, and you want to avoid spillage. Sheri had a better idea:

> An elegant older lady had a buttock tuck done at our office. She is richer than God, as proper as she is nice, and a very fastidious person. The idea of peeing into a cup was, well, offensive to her. The cup was hard to position, and awkward. A few days into her recovery she happened to walk into the garage where her chauffeur had been changing the oil in the rather antique Bentley. There she saw the solution—an oil-changing funnel, one of those plastic funnels with a long hose-like extension on the end. It was a brilliant discovery. She experimented and learned it is simple to urinate directly into the toilet using this handy-dandy device. She shared her discovery with us, and now we tell everyone to pee through this kind of a funnel.

You can also now order a funnel made specifically for this purpose. It's called "Lady J" and costs only $6.85 from Magellan's at 1-800-962-4943. Another product that looks promising is Brief Relief, a disposable funnel-shaped container. It retails at $9.85 for a package four.

However, Sheri points out, we still have one more routine problem after a buttock tuck: How do we sit on the toilet for a bowel movement? She explains that you roll up towels into logs and build yourself a ramp against the back of the toilet so you can recline against the tank and not put any pressure on your very sore, very unbending butt.

As you heal, the skin will start to stretch and soon you will be able to bend. After a week you should be able to drive. After

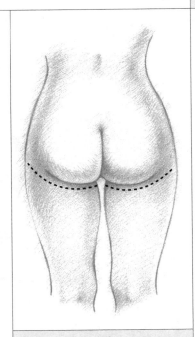

Thighplasty

three weeks you can go back to exercising. Of course, you will be wearing "the garment" (see pages 55–57). Keep it on day and night for the first week. Remember, the more compression you maintain, the better your results will be.

The "bottom" line? The benefit of a buttock tuck is a beautiful butt. The trade-off is your butt will have two long scars across its bottom, which can be easily hidden and should fade to a pencil-thin line.

- Thighplasties (there are several types) pull up the skin on the front and sides of your legs and the upper inside of your thigh.

Sheri had both a buttock tuck and thighplasty done at one time. She came out fine, but her surgeon has since decided that the operations must be done in separate procedures. There is too much tension on the incision, and, for ease of recovery, you need one side of your body healed before you do the other. Also, Sheri pushed herself too much. Soon she wasn't feeling well, and thought she was coming down with the flu. She felt achy. Her skin hurt to the touch. She began running a fever. The problem turned out to be an abscess along the incision in her groin area. With treatment the infection cleared up quickly, and her incision healed beautifully. Despite the complication, Sheri is flying high with her results. Her legs look fantastic.

The benefits of a thighplasty are undimpled, beautifully contoured thighs. The trade-off? A scar at the very top of your leg and probably extending into the groin area.

- Bra bulge and brachioplasty. We hate bingo arms! And we moan about our bra bulge, that bulge of flesh and fat that sticks out next to our armpits when we wear a bra. Unfortunately, liposuction alone won't give you perfect results. The skin is thin here and the fat is soft—so retraction might be a problem. Just sucking away the fat of bingo arms might also leave you with some loose skin. If that happens, you will need a brachio-plasty—a procedure which cuts away the excess skin and leaves you with beautifully contoured biceps and triceps, and unfortunately, a scar.

OUR FINAL WORD

Girlfriends, we can't stress strongly enough that each of the procedures in this section—liposuction, abdominoplasty, and the nips and tucks discussed in this chapter—has a trade-off. The benefits are often dramatic, beautiful, and rejuvenating. But with liposuction you may have bumps, lumps, and loose skin. With tummy tucks and other skin-reduction surgeries, you will have scars. You need to weigh the benefits against the losses. Fortunately, advances in this field are being made quickly. A few years

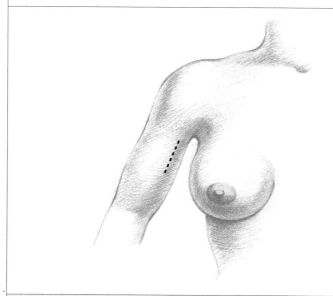

brachioplasty

ago, performing surgeries that left noticeable scars seemed out-of-date, when the technology was moving toward making tiny incisions. But women demanded help; they made it clear they would gladly accept the trade-offs to get rid of disfiguring, redundant skin.

For many of us, the trade-off is worth it.

ALL ABOUT BOOBS

5

"Tits on a Stick:" Breast Augmentation

The trip to Hooterville begins with words like these (and all were uttered by girlfriends we know):

- "I want to look like Pamela Anderson."
- "I just want what the children took away."
- "I really don't want to be bigger; I just want what I used to have."
- "I want perky."
- "I just want to feel good in a bathing suit."
- "I never want to see another Wonderbra."
- "I want to burn this bra."
- "I want big. I mean *big.*"

It's the honest-to-God truth: No woman is satisfied with her breasts. We *obsess* over them. They're too big, too small, one is bigger than the other, one is higher than the other, they sag, the nipples are too big, the nipples are too small. We stand in front of the mirror for hours, staring, sighing, wishing we were different.

Sometimes, we stand in front of the mirror and cry. For many women whose childbearing has left them with "fried eggs on a nail" or "empty wet socks," the loss of the figure they once had is unbearable. They feel bad about their bodies and are miserable about their breasts.

It may not be possible to have absolutely perfect breasts. But with breast-augmentation surgery we can have bigger ones—Dolly Parton–sized if we want them (and yes, she did have implants!). Women who have been "flattened" by childbearing can have perkier breasts, or fuller ones again. In fact, for women with pancakes instead of milkshakes, breast implants, along with an operation called mastoplexy (to uplift badly sagging breasts), can remove a terrible emotional hurt. Many painful things in life we have to live with; feeling bad about our breasts is *not* one of them.

GOING BIG

Of all the cosmetic-surgery procedures, breast augmentation rates highest on the satisfaction list. In 1998, according to the American Society for Aesthetic Plastic Surgery, 126,913 women had breast augmentation. There are rarely any serious complications. In fact, the most common complaint is that women wish they had gone bigger! With the incision made in the armpit and the implant put *on top* of the muscle (many doctors don't do this), it is a nearly painless procedure that leaves a very small scar in a place nobody sees it

Note one exception to this, girlfriends: Badly sagging breasts that require an uplift will need incisions in the front of the breast. This operation is discussed in the next chapter, on breast reduction.

Now what about this "tits on a stick" business? Susan listens to hundreds of women each year, and she says this "look" is what women who come in for breast augmentation want—no hips, no ass, flat stomach, and big boobs. Look at the Playboy channel on satellite TV. Think Barbie. For better or worse, "tits on a stick" is the look of the new millennium. Now, this ideal shape is

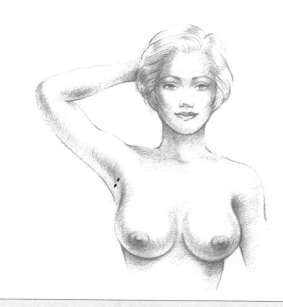

Underarm incision

probably impossible for most normal human beings to attain, but with liposuction and breast augmentation, women can come close, or at least closer.

Charlee admits,

> I didn't give the procedure much thought before I did it. That's the truth. I was having a midlife overhaul, the works. I was emotionally down and out, and over forty. My breasts fit a 34B bra, not big, but they pushed up with a push-up bra and they were "okay." In fact, they were cute breasts when I was in my twenties. I looked like a blonde Sally Field playing the Flying Nun—terminally cute. I kept my dissatisfaction with my breast size hidden away deep inside me. I never mentioned it at all. After all, from the 1970s on, it wasn't "politically correct" to want big breasts.

How small was I, really? When my older sister saw my "before" pictures, she said, "It looks as if you never finished developing." I guess that's the story of my life, unfinished development.

Well, there I was, finally going under the knife to repair what age and too-rapid weight loss had taken away (my tummy tuck) and suddenly I had this idea. I figured I had lived the first half of my life able to go braless, favoring drop-waist dresses, having nothing but air where cleavage ought to be, and generally feeling like a prepubescent kid with my clothes off. So I decided to just, as they say, *do it*. Then after seeing another girlfriend's new breasts, I decided to do it *big*. And I did.

As a result, I truly feel feminine, filled with mystery, seductive. I bend over in front of mirrors and inspect my cleavage. I strut like a majorette. And I never did realize before how much men love to look at breasts. Silly me.

Talk about instant satisfaction. I left for a trip to Europe less than two weeks after my surgery. I carried my own bags without pain or discomfort. I wore dresses cut lower than I ever dared before. A two-piece bathing suit. Tight sweaters. Latex tops (this is from a former customer of Laura Ashley, you should know). European men went bananas. In fact, there was this one incident in a lurching train through the Alps . . .

So girlfriends, if you're not ready to be looked at, stared at, gaped at, smiled at, whistled at, or have leers directed at you, and if you're not able to deal with adoring men with good humor and a happy glow, you probably don't really want to do this at all.

Face facts, girlfriends. With the exception of exotic dancers, models, and show-business hopefuls, the reason most women have breast augmentation is vanity. You may look fine to everyone else in the world but yourself. But *your feelings* are what counts. New breasts won't make a relationship better. New breasts will not bring you love. So *never, ever* get breasts to please a boyfriend, lover, or significant other (including movie producers). Change your breast size only for yourself. If you are unhappy with the breasts you have, we'll tell you what you are really getting into if you opt to get brand-new ones. Weigh *the facts* against living the fantasy; then make the best decision *for you*.

SAFETY FIRST

The biggest question women have about getting augmentation surgery is: Will the implants cause cancer or an immune disorder? Everyone has heard the horror stories about silicone implants. Are the stories true? What *are* implants made of? What risks are you taking?

First off, most of the implants in current use are filled with sterile saline solution (salt water). Saline solution is the stuff you put in your eyes if you have contacts. Surgeons use it to wash out wounds. If an implant ruptures and saline pours into your system, *nothing will happen.* (We have heard of implants rupturing only twice: one woman was in an auto accident; the other was kicked by a horse. The implants were removed through the original incision and replaced.) Your body just absorbs the saline, and you pee it out. Saline has no calories, no nutrients, is non-allergenic, and it can't hurt you in any way.

There are some new implants that are filled with vegetable oil, and silicone-filled implants are again on the market. Whatever material fills the implant, the covering is still silicone. Its real name is "medical grade silicone elastomer." Should you be concerned about the silicone covering? We know there has been controversy over silicone used in the body, so we researched it. Here's what we found:

There is no evidence that a breast implant increases your risk of getting any kind of breast tumor (Engel, 571–72). After thirty years of clinical use, there is no evidence that silicone breast implants cause cancer (Deapen, 361–68). There is no evidence that having an implant can cause birth defects (Kennedy et al: 909–20).

And now for the biggie: Can implants cause autoimmune disease or chronic fatigue, muscle pain, joint pain and swelling, arthropathy, scleroderma, lupus, Raynaud's syndrome, or rheumatoid arthritis—the kind of illnesses and mysterious pains that have sent women to court to sue? Research studies, including a recent, important Mayo Clinic study, state unequivocally that implants don't cause illness of any kind (Spiera et al, 239–45).

Significant health problems have happened to women with implants, there is no question about that. So far, however, nothing indicates that the implants caused the problem (Sanchez-Guerrero et al, 158–68). The conclusion is that the illnesses would have happened even if the woman didn't have implants. Studies have also found that if these health problems do happen, taking the implant out doesn't help (Spiera et al, 239–45).

If you still feel uneasy or want more information, ask a librarian to help you research this. Start with the articles we cite at the end of this book, or go right to the latest studies out there. Don't be afraid to ask someone with a medical background to review the literature with you. (Some of these articles are very technical and hard for anyone to understand. Don't feel you are being "dumb" if you start reading and the medical jargon suddenly sounds like gibberish.) Be sure you feel confident that you have the facts before you make your decision.

Women also are concerned about mammograms after breast augmentation (FDA, 2). Breast implants *may* complicate getting an accurate reading on your mammogram. You should reveal that you have had an implant. The literature from the FDA says that squeezing your breast flat could rupture the implant. (Susan feels this is unlikely. See her story about how tough implants are in the section below, called "Your Warranty.") The FDA also suggests a woman with implants needs to request a radiologist who is experienced in imaging breasts with implants, to look over the mammogram to get an accurate reading (FDA, 2).

Shopping for size and shape.

Let's start with the easier decision, shape. If you have ever watched any X-rated videos, strictly by accident, of course, you have probably seen some good examples of the "round" mammary implant. That's the problem—you *can* see them. They look like half a grapefruit or cantaloupe. They are very popular, and to tell the truth, some guys like the look.

A more natural-looking implant is called the "anatomical" shape. It looks so real, nobody will know for sure, except you and your doctor. Honest. You can ask your surgeon to see the implant he or she intends to use, and you can request the shape you prefer.

Predicting how new breasts will look on you.

Some surgeons let you put the implant in a bra and try it on to give you an idea of size. Don't bother. Seriously, this method is not going to work. The implant in your bra will appear much larger than the implant in your body, which spreads out under the skin.

A better way to get an idea of size is to look at pictures. Your surgeon will probably have a photo album you can look at. But remember, pictures are not three-dimensional. If you want to copy the look of some famous hooters, all Susan and Charlee can tell you is our guess is that Dolly Parton is over a 1,000cc breast size (and those babies would have to be custom-made).

In fact, as we said before, what we recommend before you make a decision on size and shape is to see the breasts of someone who has had the implant and has a shape similar to yours. *Oh no!* you may be thinking, *I couldn't do that. I couldn't ask.* Ninety-nine

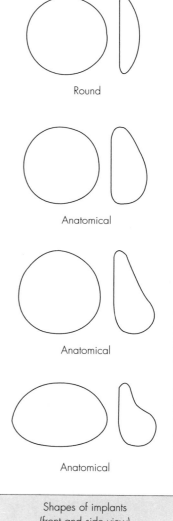

Round

Anatomical

Anatomical

Anatomical

Shapes of implants
(front and side view)

out of 101 times you won't have to. Most women who have had implants love to show them off. Previously very demure women, women so modest they refused to undress for gym class, willingly start stripping, sometimes for strangers.

Our friend Barb Gresh, never a shrinking violet, acts as what she calls a "surgical liaison." When a woman is considering breast augmentation, Barb is willing to model her "girls." The left one she named "Lola," the right one "Bambi." "I show everyone," she says. And she answers questions, too. The most common questions are: "Do you have sensation in them?" (the answer is yes) and "Do they feel like two bricks on your chest?" (the answer is no). And many women ask to feel Barb's breasts, too.

Barb has anatomical 370cc implants (they are actually 350cc implants, filled to 370cc). When a person sees them on Barb, they have an immediate opinion—either, "Oh, that's just want I want," or, "No, I don't want to be that big," or, "Gee, how about bigger?" Seeing the implant "in the flesh," so to speak, is the best way to decide on shape and size.

Age is another determinant of what size to get. Younger girl-friends may want to go smaller. Twenty-two-year-old, five-foot-eight-inch Dina had 250cc implants—small ones, especially for a taller woman like her. A beautiful young woman with long honey-brown hair, Dina had simply gotten tired of having to use "Curves" (falsies) and tape to get any kind of cleavage when she entered beauty contests. However, the adjustment of having new breasts was difficult for her. Even with the modest size of her new breasts, she still thought twice about wearing T-shirts, crop-tops, or sweaters. Often she put on a blazer to completely disguise her new size. She told no one but her immediate family and her best friend. Later, she worried about telling even that friend. She dreaded people commenting on her increased bust size, and told one friend who mentioned she looked bustier that she was wearing "Curves." The comment of a former boyfriend—"I'd break up with you in a minute if you ever did anything like [get an implant]"—lingered in mind. She worried that having implants could impact a future relationship. These are issues Dina needed to work out before she could feel comfortable with augmentation. Dina's dilemmas, however, raise important issues women should consider *before* surgery.

On the other end of the scale is forty-eight-year-old Gabrielle. When her set of five-year-old implants began to droop over time, she went to see her surgeon about an uplift. He told her that was an option, or she could replace her implants with something a bit larger, which would fill up the slack. Gabrielle, with her black-Irish looks and intense blue eyes, has a wild Celtic streak behind those career-gal clothes. She found herself saying, *Why not? But if we're going bigger, why not go biggest?* She decided on 900cc implants—and yes, she does look like Dolly Parton, with her tiny waist and very prominent breasts. She explains,

> At my age, I'm totally comfortable with my sexuality. It was disconcerting at first for men to stare so directly at my chest, but I never felt bothered or harassed. I "dress down" for work, using a suit jacket to minimize the impact of my breasts. I dress "classy" when I go out for an evening, but I do show off my cleavage. The only negative comments I've gotten were from women. I wore an elegant strapless gown to a Christmas ball, and some of them were real bitches! *Meow!* Even a good friend of mine suggested that there was something wrong with me for "doing that to myself."
>
> Look, if I get tired of these breasts—and yes, there are some negatives!—I will take them out, get smaller implants and have the uplift operation I originally wanted. Going really big was a win-win situation for me. And I feel psychologically I was ready to handle it.

Sizes of implants range from 150ccs on up to custom-made, very large models like Gabrielle's. How large do you need to go? It depends on your preference, your height, and your build. Remember two factors: (1) the shorter your torso (or the higher-waisted you are), the larger the breast is going to look; and (2) the size you end up with depends on the amount of breast tissue you started with. The implant will add to what you already have. One more important point for gals who are trying to put back what the children took away: You need to get an implant big enough to approximate the size you were before to completely fill, or overfill, the area.

Another true-life story from our files.

Before becoming a mother, Monica was a showgirl-like knockout. She had a body that earned wolf whistles! But after three children, Monica's once glorious breasts hung down to her waist. She hated the way she looked and finally decided to get breast augmentation. Unfortunately, Monica went to a surgeon who gave her a 250cc implant under the muscle. The surgery was painful, scarred her, and the results were truly a nightmare. Monica still had badly sagging breasts, only now the flaccid breast tissue drooped off the end of a strange mound-like protrusion from her chest, looking like nothing in nature should. She described the appearance of each breast as looking like a fist inserted halfway into a pair of knee-highs. Monica tearfully complained to her surgeon. He curtly told her she should be pleased with the result, that it was the best she could expect, and that nothing could be done.

Wrong, wrong, and wrong again!

Fortunately, Monica listened to girlfriends who told her to go see a different doctor. She ended up at the office of Susan's husband, our own Dr. Francis J. Collini. He proposed refilling her breasts back to the bountiful size she had once been—650ccs! Fortunately, she didn't need an uplift operation. Dr. Collini used an anatomic implant that was placed under the skin, after he removed the old implant from under the muscle. Monica still had scars, though they were well hidden under her now magnificent breasts. Her breasts looked like they once had and appeared completely natural. On Monica, although not a very tall woman, 650ccs—which are really big breasts—look great. But the sad thing is that she had to go through the expense and the physical ordeal of two surgeries.

Less is not more when it comes to deciding on size.

The most common implant in most plastic surgery practices is 250ccs. On all the women we've seen, that is a small breast. Post-op, a girlfriend will look pretty, pert, and far from flat-chested, but she often discovers that her breasts are really not as big as she envisioned—especially after the initial swelling goes down.

HAVING THE SURGERY

If you have breast-augmentation surgery with the incision made under the armpit, you can expect to be under (very light) anesthesia for two to three hours. How gory *is* the operation? Barb actually watched Charlee's surgery and said it was "fascinating," and an incredible sight—watching the implants being filled and the new breasts emerge. Talk about inflation! Because the anesthesia does not put you into a heavy sleep, Charlee—not the silent type under any circumstances—gabbed away nonstop through the entire procedure. "What did I say? I don't want to know!"

When you wake up, you will already be wearing a truly ugly flesh-colored surgical bra. Your doctor should provide it for you, having measured your chest before surgery. To tell the truth, you really need two. The first bra put on after surgery is going to get stained and bloody right under the arms. You are going to want to rinse it out, but you must keep a bra on continuously for three to four days after surgery. *Don't cheat,* girlfriends. You really need to

> ### CHOOSE WISELY— CHOOSE A LITTLE BIGGER
>
> **T**he advice we have for most of you is: Get an implant of at least 300ccs. The number one complaint of most women who have gotten breast augmentation is, "I should have gone bigger!"

wear the darned thing twenty-four hours a day. It shapes and molds your implants. So if you aren't provided with two, buy an extra one. After a week, you can wear a not-too-tight sports bra to give yourself a break from the flesh-colored monster, which some women complain bothers their incisions or chafes them under the arms where they are very sensitive.

After your breast-augmentation surgery, you will feel floaty, weak, a little disoriented, and/or groggy. Besides those feelings, you will have no desire whatsoever to move your arms more than is necessary. Some girlfriends had nausea the night after the operation. We haven't talked to anyone who got really sick or had a lot of pain.

A Girlfriend's Tip on Post-Op Clothes

Plan to have changes of clothing that do not require being slipped on over your head. This includes nighties. *No T-shirts unless they are really, really oversized!* Think about wearing clothes that do not require you to raise your arms to put on.

Post-Operative Tips and Advice

Hopefully, your surgeon will provide you with information. You might use this chapter as a basis for discussion when you speak to your surgeon. You should be thoroughly familiar with it if you plan to have implants. The more you know, the safer you are.

What to Expect Medically

- A small amount of bloody drainage for three to five days after the surgery.
- Bruising and swelling. Most women say you may have some bruising in three places: under your new breasts on your torso,

high up on your front where your breasts meet your chest (an injection site), and under your arms—how *much* bruising varies a lot from individual to individual. (Reminder: Taking vitamin E supplements increases the amount of bleeding and bruising, so you need to stop taking it before surgery—and if you have been taking it for years, stop taking it *six months in advance*.) Diligent application of ice packs, oral vitamin C, arnica montana, and vitamin K cream will speed healing. Normally, bruising is completely resolved by three weeks.

- Mild discomfort. You should *not* experience pain after this procedure. However, it is not unusual to feel brief pains for several weeks following surgery. These pains go away when the swelling does. In fact, if you have significant pain, call your doctor immediately.

- Numbness. Parts of your breasts and your nipples may be numb. This is more a nuisance than a medical problem, and

XXX-RATED INFORMATION

Boobs are part of your sexuality. They are a big attraction to men. You have been fantasizing (oh, admit it!) about lovemaking after your operation, or at least about the outfit you're going to wear in the pre-sex seduction scene—which brings up the issue of sex. For the first *two weeks* any sexual activity is *not* recommended. You are not allowed to raise your blood pressure by any means. Girlfriend, your lover may get incredibly turned on by your new boobs, but more likely, he's going to be scared to touch you. And you are going to feel about as sexual as a turnip. Many women find touching painful for *a few weeks*.

After the two weeks are up, for those of you with Fred Flintstones, tell those cavemen to be gentle or begone. Since you are not going to want any sort of pressure on your breasts when you finally "do it," you may want to try the following positions: sitting on him, missionary style (with no hugging you or using you as a mattress when he's done), doggy style, or some strange Kama-Sutra variation.

Although you may look like a *Playboy* centerfold, you might not be able to feel a thing for a while; numbness of the breasts and nipples is pretty common. Yes, it goes away (*almost* always).

feeling returns over several months. Occasionally, some diminished sensitivity may last indefinitely.

- Scars. If you have incisions under your armpits, they will first get a bit darker, then fade with time, and eventually will look like thin, fine white lines. If you have incisions under your breasts, they should be hidden most of the time.

- Hard breast texture and high contour. Your new breasts will be very high, feel hard as a volleyball, and the skin will look stretched and shiny. Rest assured that your breasts will soften and bottom out within a few weeks.

- Uneven sensitivity. One breast may be more sensitive than the other. This is normal.

- Asymmetry. Girlfriends, if your breasts weren't the same size before, don't expect them to be exactly the same afterward. Your surgeon will make every effort to get them as alike as possible, but if one nipple is a few centimeters higher than the other, chances are the two sides of your body and face are just as uneven. We talk about the body's asymmetry wherever you have two of anything in section 3, "About Face," but nobody's two boobs are identical. After surgery you are going to be scrutinizing them—and other people will scrutinize them. (There's a funny bit on that in the movie *Summer Rental* starring John Candy—rent it if you haven't seen it.) You may not have really noticed if your nipples were directly in line before the operation. Try not to get crazy about any *small* differences in symmetry.

- Heavy feeling. You *are* heavier! You have more weight on the front of your chest (from one to three pounds). This new weight can change your posture and your center of balance.

- Soreness in chest muscles. This should go away in about three to four days.

- Sloshing and rippling. This can happen with saline implants. The cause is an implant that is not fully filled. The remedy is to have the implant filled to maximum capacity.

COMPLICATIONS

There are a few complications to watch for with breast-augmentation surgery:

- Infection. This is unlikely since you will be given antibiotics, but it is always possible. Try not to contaminate the incision sites.

- Hematoma. Girlfriends, the only way you can screw this operation up is to do something really dumb. Like jogging. Or working out. Let's face it, some women are so worried about gaining weight, or so obsessive about exercise, that they might be tempted to just do "a little bit." *Don't.* We know of two women, both nurses, who went jogging the first week and ended up with hematomas (a collection of blood inside the body that may have to be surgically drained). No matter how good you feel, and most women have just minor discomfort, take it easy, and it's probably safest to avoid any heavy lifting or strenuous exercise for *a month.* If a hematoma does occur, *call your doctor.* You may need to have it evacuated (drained) in the office.

- Hypersensitivity. What "hypersensitivity" means is that, instead of being pleasurable, the sensation of being touched quickly turns painful. This can put a damper on your sex life. "Look, but don't touch!" We suggest you gently rub your nipples yourself, always stopping short of causing discomfort. Use a pleasant moisturizer or skin cream. Hopefully, your toleration of touch will come back in time.

- Capsular contraction. This, girlfriends, is the number one major medical complication with implants. In some people, for some reason scar tissue forms around the implant and the

---

WHEN TO CALL YOUR DOCTOR

- If is there is excessive bleeding or swelling.

- If you develop a fever or other signs of infection; i.e., pus at incision sites or red streaks from incision sites.

breast becomes hard and painful. There is no way to predict who will be affected. If it occurs, it is first treated with a process called "closed capsulotomy." This is done in the office, and manual compression is used to break up the scar tissue. If this fails, the problem can be fixed surgically, by opening an incision and removing the scar tissue. Sometimes the implant itself will be replaced.

The Shock of Transformation

When you wake up from the anesthesia and look down (or in a mirror) at your new breasts, don't panic. You will look very different. And what you are seeing at first is *not* an accurate picture of how you will look in a few weeks.

Very likely you may feel a tremendous anxiety about your new body image. You will think your breasts look too big—huge, even gigantic. Ninety percent of patients are truly concerned about their size when they wake up after the operation. If you start to become upset or anxious, or are suddenly overtaken by regret, take a deep breath and relax. You are normal. Remember, at first you

---

PREGNANCY AFTER BREAST AUGMENTATION

Are you worried about what will happen to your breasts if you end up pregnant after your augmentation surgery? Is it a factor in making your decision, especially if you are under forty? Here's what you need to know:

- During pregnancy your breasts will enlarge and become engorged normally, just like breasts without implants. Your implants will not be affected.

- Typically, you will be able to breastfeed. *However, there are no guarantees.* The implants will not contaminate breast milk or affect your baby's health.

- After your pregnancy, yes, you might droop. Your breasts will not become flat after your hormones return to normal—an experience some women have—but you may find you will need an uplift operation at some point.

will be very swollen. By the time the swelling and bruising resolve, you will be more comfortable with your new looks. However, the loss of the way you looked before surgery, even if you were dissatisfied with your breasts, is still a loss. You have given up a bit of who you were to gain a different figure. So if you feel a bit sad, if you feel some regret, let yourself have the feelings. Find a girlfriend who has had the operation to talk to. Express your feelings if you can. If you can't talk about them, at least acknowledge them.

Of course, you might not have those feelings at all. Many girlfriends were giddy with joy and flying with happiness when they saw their new breasts.

There is a six-month period of adjustment for breast augmentation. Like nose jobs, this procedure is connected with many emotional and psychological issues. *If you need a professional to talk to after your surgery, do it.* You may have stirred up some long-standing issues about yourself, your sexuality, and your body image.

Slow down, Superwoman.

Chances are, you are going to feel pretty good even the next day after surgery. But listen, girlfriends, take a full week off from work. If you have a desk job, yes, you can get away with going in on day four (you are supposed to keep ice packs on the tops and sides of your breasts for the first three days—and warm soaks for three more, so you really will be doing more than you should). Try not to work at all for the first week; give yourself the entire time to recover. If you try to do too much, you're going to feel cranky, maybe depressed, and totally wiped out.

Your Warranty

The FDA warns that no one knows how long the implants will last, but chances are they will have to be replaced someday. That's the bad news. The good news is that even as you are coming out of the anesthesia after your operation, you are given a "device identification card" and a lifetime implant replacement guarantee that should offer, as one company states, "lifetime replacement and limited financial reimbursement in the event of loss of product shell integrity, subject to certain conditions." I wish my car's tires came with the same deal.

How tough are breast implants? Susan tells this story:

> The husband of a patient came to see me in my office to discuss "a problem." He was afraid to touch his wife's breasts for fear of breaking the implants. He wanted to know how strong the material really was. I had an implant filled with saline available to show patients. First I took it and wrung it like you would wring out a towel. Then I threw it on the floor and stomped on it—*bam, bam, bam.* Last, I took it and lobbed it with all my strength (and I have a great throwing arm) against the wall of my office. The implant remained unharmed.
>
> The man stood there with his mouth agape. "I guess you can give your wife a little squeeze now and then," I said.

The high and the mighty.

How will you feel in the first weeks after the operation? One girl-friend said, "I feel like my breasts are sitting on my shoulders." That's what everybody feels like. For the weeks right after surgery, your new breasts are going to be very full on top. You may feel puffed out right up to the collarbone. The skin may be stretched so tight that it's shiny. The common description from women who have had children is that they felt "engorged."

Our girlfriend Danielle wanted to know how long her breasts would feel hard. The answer is, you will begin to notice a difference after a week, and the swelling and fullness will steadily disappear.

After three months you will find that your breasts have dropped a bit, are softer, and have become somewhat smaller than they were right after the operation.

Because of that change, your doctor usually advises you not to run out and buy a new bra. We say, Oh, go on! Make that trip to Victoria's Secret. There is a chance you'll have to buy another size later. But unless you're really watching your budget, we say, "Splurge!" You have been waiting for this moment. Enjoy buying a non-padded, non-uplift, gorgeous, sexy bra that is a size C, D . . . or even DD. When Charlee went shopping for a sports bra she could do aerobics in, it was an incredible thrill to buy a bra for "a bigger-breasted woman." "Bigger-breasted"? You'll suddenly realize, *That's me!*

Another common reaction is that most women keep looking at themselves as they assume myriad positions: straight down, by tilting their head and seeing new cleavage; in the mirror, frontal view; in the mirror, side view; chest inflated; chest relaxed. This surgery brings hours of fun posing naked and in various garments.

Clothes for the full-figured gal.

As you are soon to find out, at least half your wardrobe will have made its last appearance on your body the day you go in for breast augmentation. Say good-bye graciously to that very expensive, very tight little leather jacket; that beautiful bustier, size 32A; the cute little jumper with no waist; anything A-line—*all your bras.*

Therefore another expense you need to consider is a new wardrobe. Some of your pre–big-boob clothes won't button, will gap if they do, or simply will not—like your old bras—go on at all. Other clothes, from outerwear to undies, will not be flattering. Waistless dresses, which used to make you look charming or cute, will now give you the shape of, well, a refrigerator. Boxy, unfitted jackets or blazers will make you look fat or—oh, God—matronly. A-lines will look as if your wardrobe was designed by

Ahab the tentmaker. And those darling empire-waist sundresses? You will, um, look pregnant.

You may have to try on styles you never considered before to discover what flatters your new assets. In general, you need clothes that are very fitted to show off your waistline and flatter your bust-line. Maybe you need to check out those old Marilyn Monroe movies, or notice that Dolly Parton's country-western shirts have darts to pull in the fabric under her colossal, classic hooters. You can become a sweater girl, as long as you avoid oversized sweaters (or extra-large sweatshirts—you'll look like a tank). You need *snug*. Think Lycra . . . plunging necklines. For intimate nights look at the Frederick's of Hollywood catalog. Go, girlfriend!

Also, you will be entering the great uncharted land of hunting for a bra that truly fits. The bigger you are, the harder they are to find. And when you do find them, they may be . . . ugly. With implants you are supposed to avoid underwire bras. You don't want too-skinny straps that might leave indentations on your shoulders. You will have to hunt for a good bra. There are a few Victoria's Secret styles that will work. Be sure you look for ones that fit a D cup (their C cup is rather small).

Learning a new body language.

Other girlfriends have shared the following changes in lifestyle and habits:

- You may not be able to see your waist to buckle a belt or jeans. Most girlfriends can still see their feet.

- You may not feel comfortable sleeping on your stomach anymore—and in any event you *can't* for the first few weeks after surgery.

- Watch out for poor posture, especially standing stoop-shouldered. This is likely to happen when you feel tired. These babies are heavy. Gabrielle, with her 900cc implants, had a real problem with this. You really have to stay conscious of keeping your shoulders back.

- A golfer girlfriend said the boobs changed her golf swing. Tennis players may experience a similar problem.

- Jogging is difficult for some girlfriends. If so, try the Title 9 Sports Catalog Company's Frog Bra (1-800-609-0092).

WANNA SEE?

Now we want to prepare you for what seems to be a universal phenomenon. In the first few months after surgery, you are going feel a compulsion to show everybody your boobs. Okay, right now you're thinking, *I'd never.* But afterward, you'll discover you think of your implants differently than your natural breasts. They don't seem part of your body; they're more like a new pair of glasses. Chances are, you will be very excited. You lose all sense of modesty or shame. Unless you're keeping the operation a deep secret, you're going to be telling everybody.

Susie, one of the world's most genteel and demure Junior League ladies, greeted Charlee a few days after her implant surgery by squealing, "Wanna see?"—whipping off her sweater, unhooking her bra, and baring all. Nobody can get Barb to keep her clothes on, and Charlee will never confess to this, but we suspect something shocking happened with the twenty-three-year-old lawn boy.

Beware the green-eyed monster.

One last note on breast augmentation. As with other cosmetic-surgery procedures, if you get good results, prepare for some "friends," and many relatives, to be jealous. You know you look good. You made the decision after careful consideration. You did it for you. Don't let yourself be upset or put down by people who do not approve and who judge you. (Think about this beforehand.

Your supercritical aunt Rose may not be on the list of people who should know about your operation. In fact, she should never know. Let her suspect all she wants to. You can tell her you started taking hormones and, Oops, look what happened.) You may overhear remarks about your breasts being "fake" or "not yours." Your breasts *are* "real." A padded bra is "not real." (And by the way, does the catty person who spoke about your breasts color her hair or get a permanent wave?) The breasts definitely belong to you. Your new breasts will look so natural that no one who isn't told about your operation will ever guess you have an implant.

When you've got it—flaunt it. Let the naysayers eat their hearts out. You have the very best breasts money can buy.

6

Too Much of a Good Thing: Breast Reduction and Uplift

Perky, youthful breasts may seem like an impossible dream. They're not. Thanks to improved techniques, breast-reduction (mammoplasty) and breast-uplift (mastopexy) operations can radically change your shape, from hanging water balloons to gorgeous, high tits. For pouter-pigeon–breasted women—44 DD and beyond—this procedure can turn a girlfriend from matronly to "Zowie!" and provides health benefits too. For girlfriends left with sagging breasts and pancakes after childbearing, an uplift, often combined with an implant, can boost self-esteem as well as boost boobs.

The Bad Things Big Breasts Can Do

Oversized breasts cause a variety of medical problems, including

- back pain
- neck pain
- headache
- shoulder pain, and grooving (from your bra straps)
- intertrigo (a rash under the breast)

- lordosis (arthritis of the cervical spine)

- dorsal kyphosis (postural change due to a humpback)

- numbness of the outer two fingers (due to ulnar nerve compression)

- breathing difficulties

- anxiety and embarrassment, plus the inability to find bras, swimsuits, and clothes that fit on both your top and bottom.

What the procedure is like.

One of the most common techniques is called a "brassiere-pattern skin reduction." Tissue and skin is taken from the bottom of your breast and your nipple and areola are relocated, but not detached. The advantage of leaving the "stem" intact—also called the "inferior pedicle" technique of breast-reduction surgery—is that you will retain sensation and use of the nipple. Some other procedures for extremely large breasts do detach the nipple (the "free-nipple graft"), and women may have emotional difficulty with the loss of a normal, full-service nipple.

Every year surgeons are developing better techniques, and the movement is for "minimal-incision breast surgery" (Slavin, 361–69). At the current state of the art, the incisions for breast reduction or uplift may be L-shaped, J-shaped, or even an inverted T—but they are still substantial in size. See the drawing on page 117.

Doctors can also reduce the size of the areola (the dark pink-brown area circling the nipple). While there is a great variation in the size of areolas, very large ones can measure three or more inches across, and most women want them smaller. Also, among Asians, the small nipple and areola is a symbol of a sensual woman. More and more small-breasted Asian girlfriends are asking for breast augmentation *with* a nipple and/or areola reduction. This is possible with a technique called the "inner-doughnut incision" (Lai, 1695).

ALERT ON BREAST-FEEDING

The "free nipple graft" technique eliminates the possibility of breast-feeding in the future. But breast-feeding *may* or *may not* be impaired after the "inferior pedicle" technique. In other words, there are no guarantees, but it is entirely *possible* to breast-feed after a breast reduction as long as the nipple is left attached.

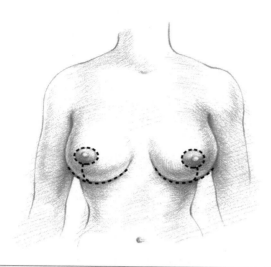

breast reduction and uplift incisions

Where the surgery is performed.

Although breast reduction is usually performed in a hospital or an outpatient surgical setting under general anesthesia, it can be done under local anesthetic and intravenous sedation. If a fear of general anesthesia is holding you back, talk it over with your doctor and express your fears. It is important to talk about them!

An uplift is usually performed under local anesthesia and intravenous sedation, but fewer procedures of either type are being done in the hospital setting. More often they are done in the surgeon's office facility. The operation for breast reduction can take from three to five hours.

Recovery from Breast Reduction and Uplift

Post-op tips and suggestions are nearly identical to those for breast augmentation, as is some of what to expect medically. But there are differences! For instance, since there are larger incisions in both breast-reduction and -uplift surgery, care of these incisions should be added to your regimen. Sutures are usually removed in about seven days.

Also, you should wear a special bra for four to six weeks after the surgery. J. C. Penney has a sports bra that provides both support and produces a satisfactory contour for the breasts. Ask your surgeon what he or she recommends—but you *must* wear one.

How long should you take off from work? Two weeks. Sure, you may feel terrific and want to go back sooner. But surgery always takes more out of you than you anticipate, from feeling "blah" to being cranky, to flat-out exhaustion. Also, you should always plan on giving yourself time to heal from complications even though chances are, you won't have any. Two weeks is optimal before going back to an outside job or resuming heavy-duty housework!

What to Expect Medically After Surgery

- Scars: The scars on the breasts look good immediately after surgery, but after four to six weeks, they begin to "mature" and become red and thickened. They can stay this way for several months to a year, when they finally lighten and soften. Some women require silicone gel sheeting or gel ointment to quicken the maturation process. This gel is worn twelve hours a day for four months and helps to soften the scar at a more rapid rate.

- Swelling and soreness: It's normal.

- Bottoming out: Breast reduction will not prevent sagging of the breasts over time. Sagging is caused by stretching of the ligaments that hold the breasts up. Also, as time passes after a breast reduction, most patients develop a "bottoming out" of the breast to one degree or another. That means the breast tissue falls downward below the nipple and the nipple migrates upward. To prevent this complication, your surgeon might make the distance between the lower end of the areola and the breast crease no greater than four centimeters, and it almost always makes this problem minimal.

COMPLICATIONS

Remember, girlfriends, the body can't be fixed like a washing machine. Everyone heals differently and lots of things can go wrong. If they do, don't panic. Work with your surgeon and most of them can be corrected. Here are some complications that can occur with breast reduction or uplift.

- Keloid or hypertropic scars. Some women, especially women of color, are prone to keloids. You probably already have a good idea if you are.

- Bleeding. It is rare for someone to bleed so much they require a transfusion, but to be on the safe side, if your pre-surgical tests

A SCARY DISCOVERY THAT COULD SAVE YOUR LIFE

All patients above the age of thirty-five, any woman with a family history of breast cancer, and any with breast nodules you can feel, will be sent to get a mammogram before surgery. *All* breast-reduction patients will receive a mammogram four to six months *after* the surgery to establish a baseline for future mammographic breast-cancer screening. This is done because fat necrosis (dead fat) and/or calcifications may develop in reduced breasts, leading to a false-positive mammogram. The baseline mammogram will keep you from being scared to death unnecessarily when your results come back.

However, all breast tissue removed during surgery is sent for pathological analysis. If an unsuspected breast cancer is found, the plastic surgeon will refer you to a surgical oncologist for evaluation and treatment. Be assured, a mastectomy will *never* be performed at the same time as the breast reduction. You never have to be afraid of waking up without a breast.

But if you have a hidden cancer, your breast-reduction surgery will find it . . . and that's a very *good* thing.

show you have a clotting problem, you may be asked to donate a unit of your own blood before the surgery.

• Loss of nipple and/or areola area. This complication is very rare. Women at greatest risk are those who are obese with very large breasts or women who do not stop smoking.

• Asymmetry of breast size. If your breasts were different sizes before surgery, they might still be afterward. The surgeon will make them as identical as he can, but it may not be possible! If the asymmetry is severe or very upsetting to you, you may be able to opt for another procedure (but don't expect it to be free!).

• Skin loss at the T-junction of the incision. The T-junction lies at the lower part of the vertical incision made just under the nipple-areola area.

  Most of the tension placed on the incision stitches is at this spot. Some doctors leave a special stitch at this location for two or three weeks after surgery to help keep it closed. Should this complication occur, it probably will heal on its own, leaving only a slight, reddish purple discoloration. (You can lighten this later with a cosmetic bleaching cream available through your doctor.)

• Nipple inversion. This is *very* rare, but it is possible that scar tissue can develop in such a way that the nipple inverts and turns inward. It can be corrected.

• Other possible complications include infection, hematoma, seroma, swelling, bruising, postoperative nausea/vomiting and/or headache, pulmonary embolism, epidermal cyst formation from remnants of the skin left on the dermal nipple-areola complex pedicile, suture rejection or "spitting" from the incision, numbness . . . and one that girlfriend Pearl got—an allergic reaction to the surgical tape!

Relief—blessed relief!

First of all, you may not have thought of this, but getting rid of your super-big bra size will take years off your appearance! You will look younger as well as thinner.

Starting with your nightclothes, you will notice inches of extra room. Get on the scale. You just lost pounds. Clean out your closet and toss those matronly jackets and dresses. Feel how your step and torso are lighter. Look in the mirror. Your shape is terrific. All the tight little jackets, cute drop-waist dresses, and other clothes the augmentation girls gave to the Salvation Army, you can now consider, although chances are, you are still well-endowed. With very few common complications, a quick recovery period, and nearly instant gratification, a breast reduction or uplift is an uplift for your spirit as well.

By and large, the biggest group of girlfriends who are totally thrilled and supremely happy about their surgery are the breast-reduction patients. Like Pearl, their only regret is that they didn't do it years earlier.

The trade-off.

You probably guessed this one: The negative that goes with this operation is scarring. Sometimes incisions heal beautifully and you are left with just a faint white line. But some scars, particularly the ones going horizontally on your breasts, have a tendency to become hypertropic (raised) or form a keloid. However, the overall improvement in the appearance of the breast is usually so dramatic that, even with the scars, the rate of satisfaction with a breast reduction or uplift is very high.

A Final Word About Cost

Insurance companies will sometimes pay part or all of the cost of breast-reduction surgery. If you have a history of any of the medical

"I had two and a half pounds removed from my right breast, three pounds from my left. A week after my operation I picked up a five-pound bucket of Sam's Club chocolate-chip cookie dough, and thought, Wow, this is heavy, maybe I shouldn't lift it. Then it hit me. I had had more than that taken off my chest!

Prior to my mammoplasty [breast reduction] I had been going to massage therapy three times a week for a stiff neck. I was plagued by chronic migraines. I had back problems. I never had a bra that fit. All those things are no longer a part of my life. I can wear a normal D-cup bra—from Victoria's Secret. I have clothes that fit. And I am pain-free. My only regret is that I didn't get a breast reduction years ago. Following my surgery, I encouraged two friends to go for consultations. They did. My advice? Do it."

PEARL, TEACHER,
AGE FORTY-TWO

problems we listed earlier, you have a better chance of being covered. One girlfriend, Mary Ann, noted that she applied toward the end of the year to her HMO and was denied. An insider tipped her off that this was because her deductible for the year was paid. She was told to reapply in the new year. She did, and was approved.

THANKS FOR THE MAMMARIES

Girlfriends, big or small, our breasts are intrinsically tied to our sexuality. Our feelings about our breasts are important and should not be belittled, by ourselves or others. If you are contemplating an augmentation, uplift, or reduction, find a supportive ally to help you through it. As we say in chapter 16 "Secrets, Lies, or Full Disclosure": "Ain't nobody's business but my own." You, and you alone, have the power and the right to make changes in your body. No one should talk you into—or out of—breast surgery. Become informed, do your homework, weigh your options, and make the very best decision for *you*. Wanting bigger breasts is not "silly" or "vain." For girlfriends with very small, uneven, or deformed breasts, augmentation can be a life-transforming procedure. And opting to reduce overly large breasts that hamper movement and affect your health is just plain sensible.

Remember the signature song of the famous French chanteuse Edith Piaf, the "Little Sparrow": *"Non, je ne regrette rien"* ("No, I regret nothing"). Girlfriends, don't look back. Make the wisest choices you can and then . . . regret nothing.

ABOUT FACE

7

Mirror, Mirror . . . Reflecting on Face-Lifts

"Doctor, only you can take my pain away," Denise's soft voice and big warm brown eyes pleaded with her plastic surgeon.

Ten years before, Denise Zawilla had been a surgical nurse, working in the operating room in a Wilkes Barre, Pennsylvania, hospital. One day during her shift in the OR, she picked up a tray of instruments, as she had done a thousand times before, and turned, twisting her back. So began ten years of unrelenting, excruciating back pain that took away not only her career, but her peace of mind. About 150 pounds at the time of her injury, she now weighed just 102. She appeared delicate and fragile. She had gone through four back surgeries, and yet the pain was still unremitting. Fearing she was becoming addicted to painkillers, she had stopped taking them. Instead Denise was coping as best she could with ceaseless pain.

A few months before seeing a plastic surgeon, Denise had been in Florida to see her mother and father. Her mother, whom Denise calls her best friend, had said to her, "Denise, I've known you've been in pain all these years, but I never could see how awful it was before. Now I see it in your eyes, and it's written all over your face."

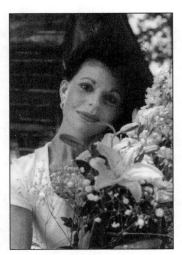

Denise Zawilla looks like a movie star following her "mini" face-lift, Alloderm, and cheek implants.

Denise was shocked. If one characteristic of her personality had always shone through, it was her upbeat nature. Energetic, funny, quick with a one-liner, she thought she had been successful at keeping her suffering from the world; even though the mirror told her every day that the constant pain and accompanying stress were aging her, she had never admitted how much. She had developed deep crow's-feet around her eyes, and bags, lines, and dark shadows under them. She laughingly called her nasolabial folds (the cleft between your nose and the outer corner of your lips) "the Grand Canyons." She had lines around her lips, too, from holding her mouth tensely. Denise was only forty-two years old. Until her mother bluntly told her what she already knew in her heart, she had never let herself voice aloud a thought that had been growing inside her: *Maybe I should have a face-lift.*

She made up her mind to have a consultation with a plastic surgeon. Together, she and her doctor decided to do a "mini" face-lift, which means only the lower portion of her face would be lifted, not her brow, not her neck. He would perform laser surgery to get rid of the lines around her eyes. The nasolabial folds, which were extremely pronounced on Denise's small face, would be a challenge. They decided to put in AlloDerm implants (see page 219) during the procedure to further "plump up" the area.

Her mom and dad came up from Florida to be with her after her surgery. Denise had prepared her mother for what she'd look like right after the operation when her head was covered in bandages. "Mom, I'm going to look like a plane-crash victim," she cautioned.

Her recovery was uncomplicated and easy.

I'm not the type of person who walks by a mirror and stares at myself, but every day I found myself looking, amazed at the constant improvement and the changes. Okay, at first you look like you went through a car windshield. You improve rapidly. I hate being cooped up, and bruised as I was, I had to go out. I had total strangers walking up to me, saying, "Did someone beat you?" "Oh yes," I'd answer, "my boyfriend is a monster. Look what he did to me . . ." And I'd just go on and on with whatever came into my head. I can't help it, I'm just tooo bad!

Is it vain to alter, lift, or otherwise change your face?

Over one hundred thousand women had face-lifts in 1998—and the number is increasing every year, according to the American Society for Aesthetic Plastic Surgery. Many thousands also had other kinds of facial surgery to change their appearance.

Is it vain to change what God gave you? No.

Want to hear what the experts say? Girlfriends, read this:

In most human relationships, the face represents the most important expression between people. It reflects our personality and emotions and is intimately connected with both verbal and nonverbal communication. The head and face are commonly considered to be the location of "self." Because of this psychological and social significance, anything that appears abnormal in the face has a direct influence on one's self-confidence (Hage, 1799).

The verdict of the experts is: A flaw with your face, including those caused by age, is serious psychological business. Contemporary American society fully accepts and, in fact, *expects* us to correct crooked teeth, crossed eyes, or even jug ears. So why shouldn't you correct any other facial flaw that has been causing you inner pain for too many years of your life? Stop the emotional hurting. Go see a doctor for a consultation and find out what is involved in fixing it.

But what if there are no real flaws? What if you just want to be beautiful? Is that "wrong" of you? Is it really possible for surgery to transform your looks? Should you even try?

"A flaw of the spirit
Cannot be hidden on a face
But a flaw of a face
If one fixes it,
Can put a spirit right."

JEAN COCTEAU

The choices you make about your face are *your* choices. Women routinely spend a fortune on makeup and other "beauty enhancers" that aren't effective. So, if you are not satisfied with the way you look . . . if you are psychologically healthy (let's not mince words here, you know the state of your mental health; i.e., whether you are coping well with life, if you have a drug or alcohol problem, or if you are on medication for depression or anxiety)—and if you have the money, time, and burning desire—*yes,* cosmetic surgery can probably make you beautiful, on the outside, at least. On the inside, it's up to you.

Is there an advantage to being good-looking in our society? You bet your sweet bippie. Like it or not, and all *"shoulds"* aside, there have been numerous studies showing what experience has already told you: Being beautiful will open doors (Sarwar, 1139). Again, what you make of the opportunity is up to you.

But let's face it, the reason most of us get facial surgery is to turn back the clock. The years affect us all, and they show on our face in all the same ways. We get chicken neck or turkey wattles; bulldog jowls, basset-hound eyes, marionette mouth, and maybe a permanent scowl between our eyebrows. At what age these changes happen depends on several factors—from genetics to life circumstance to overall health—but they often start after you turn thirty.

The question is: Are you happy about accepting these changes?

Is it time?

Tell the truth. Are you already fighting aging? Ask yourself: Do you feel comfortable about going out without makeup? Do you cover the gray in your hair? Are you spending significant money on moisturizers, "face-lifts in a jar," and concealing cosmetics? Did you run out and buy that product hyped for the "midlife" face—you know, the pink stuff? Do you use alpha-hydroxy products?

Have you changed the way you dress, adding more turtlenecks and scarves to cover up lines or loose skin on your neck? When you look in the mirror, are your eyes immediately drawn to the areas you most want to conceal? Have you surreptitiously pulled up on the skin at the side of your face just to see how you'd look with a little nip and tuck?

When you go to a family gathering, do older relatives coo, "Oh, you look just like your mother"? Maybe people at work have remarked that you look tired when you're not, or sad, when you're not, or grumpy, when you're not. Maybe you've been passed by on the job for someone younger and "more energetic."

Now, girlfriends, let's be very blunt and put out in the open other things you may be noticing. Have men stopped looking at you, or flirting? Are you becoming "invisible" in department stores, at parties, or other public places? Are you wearing your hems longer, your clothes more matronly, and not wearing some beautiful outfits you really like because they'd look "too young" on you? Most of all, have your looks stopped matching the person you feel you are inside? That's what many girlfriends have said: Their exterior didn't match their mental image of themselves.

TAKE THE TEST

If you are toying with the idea of a face-lift, and wondering if it's time, try this "objective" examination.

Begin by looking at your eyes. Do you have bags or dark circles under them? Perhaps you are starting to get little ridges or wrinkle lines below your eyes and over your cheekbones. Are you using concealer makeup or highlighter on a regular basis? Once you put on your eyeshadow, can you see it, or does your lid disappear under a droop of skin? Do your eyes give you the appearance of being tired all the time?

If you see these very first signs of aging, and the rest of your face still looks quite youthful, you can get surgery specifically on your eyes. It's called a blepharoplasty (see pages 150–59). One plastic-surgery nurse said this is what she advises for anyone who doesn't want to spend a fortune, wants a short recovery time, but wants to see a significant change in the way she looks.

But for many girlfriends, just doing your eyes isn't enough. They are just one symptom of aging among several others written on your face.

What are the unmistakable "others"? Here's the rest of your self-test.

1. Lift up your bangs or push your hair off your forehead. Do you have horizontal lines? Are there vertical lines or "frown" lines between your eyes? Do your eyebrows seem lower than they used to be? Are they beginning to droop on the outer edges?

   If you answered yes to any of these questions, you may be a candidate for a brow-lift alone, or as part of a full face-lift.

2. Look at the middle of your face, between your cheekbone and mouth. Do you have creases or lines along the top of your cheekbones? Or do you have pronounced nasolabial grooves (those depressions that go from the edge of your nose to the corner of your lips)? A deep groove adds years to your looks. Do the fattest parts of your cheeks seem to have "fallen" or have your cheeks sunk at all? These are all signs of midface laxity. A face-lift can help.

3. Look at yourself in profile. Is your neck sagging under the chin—or is there a little paunch of fat there? Can you see "rings of Venus" around your neck? And what is the skin like on your neck? Is it bumpy like that of a plucked chicken?

   Then, notice if you still have a youthful curve to your jawline, or is there a "corner" or sag? Nothing will make you look more middle-aged than jowls and a sagging neck. And they are impossible to hide. A face-lift can make them disappear completely, and restore a completely youthful profile.

4. Now for the real moment of truth. Put a mirror on a table and bend over it to see yourself. Does the flesh fall forward, surrounding your eyes, giving you chipmunk cheeks, and looking like it has come loose from the bones underneath? You don't have to be middle-aged, either, because this laxity starts happening *in your thirties,* or even earlier. If your face "falls" a lot, it's time to get a full facial lift!

Girlfriend Rosemary C. had a wonderful metaphor for when it's time to get surgery: "Before my face-lift surgery, I felt like a rumpled, unmade bed. I just didn't feel neat and well-groomed. That's important to me because I'm a business owner. Now I know I look my best."

Four Myths that Keep Girlfriends from Having a Face-Lift

Myth 1: "My face will look masklike or pulled." New techniques have eliminated the "sucked through a wind tunnel" look some people still associate with face-lifts. The platysma cervical lift (PCL) is a newer procedure, perfected over the past decade by surgeons in Sweden, Mexico, and the United States, and specifically designed to

PORE IT OUT!

Have you started obsessing about the size of your pores? Do they seem to be getting larger? Actually three things are happening. First, as your skin loses elasticity and starts sagging, your pores do elongate a bit. Second, they appear bigger because of the way they are catching the light. Because of sagging skin, the edges of your pores will cast a tiny shadow, making you notice the pores more. Third, when dead cells and sebum (oil) fill up a pore, they push the walls of the pore apart. When these pores are cleaned out with a glycolic-acid product, the walls of the pore collapse inward, and the pore will look smaller. Other resurfacing techniques (laser, peels, and dermabrasion) will also make your skin look smoother and more refined But the most satisfying results—and the best pore "shrinkage"—will come from restoring the smooth contours and tautness of your skin with a lift.

produce a more natural appearance after surgery. It minimizes the "tip-offs" that give away the fact that a face-lift has been done. Instead of simply pulling the facial skin back, the PCL sculpts the internal framework of the face, tightening sagging facial muscles and eliminating the sagging of the neck. Surgeons are able to create a completely natural look, even with second and third face-lifts.

Myth 2: "The recovery will take too long. I can't miss work." Recovery from a face-lift is extremely short, not long! Most women feel completely comfortable resuming all normal social activities in ten days. With vitamin K cream and arnica montana speeding up the healing of bruises, you can probably go out in three or four days. You can use a pair of sunglasses to hide the redness under your eyes (from a lower-lid blepharoplasty if you have one with the lift), and arrange your hair to cover the incisions in front of your ears. A scarf around your neck or high collar will hide any bruising there. And, girlfriends, here are two surefire cover stories if anyone asks, "What happened to you?"

> I had dental surgery. All four wisdom teeth had to be pulled. I was under for hours!

> I had a minor car accident and the air bag went off. Slammed me right in the face. What an ordeal! I was wearing glasses and it pushed them right into my nose. I have two black eyes, but nothing's broken, thank goodness! I'm just bruised.

If you are determined no one should know, book a hotel room out of town for three weeks and enjoy yourself. You can come home looking great and honestly say what a difference getting away can make!

Myth 3: "I'm afraid of the pain." Girlfriends, there is little or no pain with a PCL face-lift. Honest to God. You are numb, especially along the sides of your face. This eventually goes away (nerves heal slowly, so it takes a long time). But the benefit of the numbness is that nothing hurts. Most girlfriends said nothing was even sore. Some girlfriends had a headache the day after surgery. Most never took a pain pill. You do look pretty awful for the first twenty-four hours, but you don't feel a thing.

Myth 4: "Face-lifts" are too expensive. I can never afford one." Can you afford a vacation? A new car? A living-room suite? A riding lawnmower? "Oh," you say, "you can take out a loan or use a credit card for those things." Girlfriends, heed what Teresa said of her cosmetic surgery: "This is my home improvement." Start a savings club, use a credit card, take out a loan, but you can afford a face-lift if you want it.

What age do you want to be?

Patients perceived themselves as looking an average 9.31 years younger following the primary surgery [first face-lift], as compared to 10.19 years younger following second [face-lift] surgery (Guyuron, 1281).

Girlfriends, how much younger you look after surgery is largely a matter of choice, your physical condition, and the surgeon's skill. As the quote above says, most women look about ten years younger. Angie, a seventy-three-year-old great-grandmother, looks appropriate for her age—If her age were sixty! She started out with eyelid surgery ten years ago, a face-lift five years ago, and then had a brow-lift and cheek implants. What does "appropriate" mean? Angie looks like a vibrant, healthy, mature woman. She doesn't look like an old woman with a young face. The biggest visual effect of her facial surgeries has been to make her look well-groomed, elegant, and most of all, filled with life.

Speaking of men, love, and face-lifts, seeing Anna Maria today, you would never guess she's had a face-lift. But she did—and love was behind it all. Or maybe love and cheating. . . .

Married fifteen years, with two children, Anna Maria was hit broadside when a "friend" called with this bombshell: "My husband told me and made me swear not to tell. But the wife is always the last to know. So I'm telling you for your own good. Your husband is having an affair with Miss X, a former *Penthouse* model." When the shock wore off, Anna Maria found two ideas had grown out of her feelings of betrayal and anger, and they were the thoughts of a true survivor: One was a determination to look as good, and better than this blonde bimbo, this man-stealer, this "other woman." The second, just in case Anna Maria found herself divorced and dating again, was to look good enough to compete in the singles scene. Even though Anna Maria was blessed with good looks, crying for months had taken its toll. She saw the strain in her face; she saw the aging accelerate. She calmly assessed the situation and made her plan: to get a face-lift.

After she had her lift, Anna Maria remembers,

No matter how sad I felt, I'd get up in the morning and go into the bathroom. There I'd see myself in the mirror without makeup—no signs of tears, no drawn look, no sadness showing. Damn, I looked fabulous. *At least,* I'd think to myself, *even if my marriage is on the rocks, I look like a million bucks.* And then I'd feel better.

Sometimes I'd be going in to work with a heavy heart. My office was one flight up. Climbing the stairs was an effort; my legs felt like they would barely move. Everyone there knew what happened to me because in my small town, the gossip had spread like wildfire. Everyone would be staring to see how I was handling the situation today and thinking: *Is she still falling apart? Will she be able to do her job?* Right at the top of the stairs is a mirror. I'd get to the top stair and suddenly see myself. Reflected would be an impeccably made-up, glowing woman, looking stunning. Right away, I'd hold my head up, put back my shoulders, and stride into the main room where all the girls were at work. I'd have a big smile on my face because I knew, with the added help of my face-lift, I could get through this. "Good morning," I'd sing out, in a strong, happy voice. I felt I would be okay. I *was* okay. And the more cheerful I looked to the world, the more I forgot the ache in my heart.

But changes in appearance after a face-lift can be more extreme. Charlee is one example of dramatic results. Young-looking throughout her life, she discovered that in one year, the jowls she'd been dreading had appeared, her neck had gone south with a vengeance, and suddenly, there in the mirror staring back at her was . . . the spitting image of her mom. How much did Charlee's face-lift turn back the clock? Well, let's not give away all our secrets—but she ended up looking thirty, tops. Her plastic surgeon shook his head when he saw her for her three month follow-up, and laughed, "You look like a schoolgirl." And girlfriends, she did.

But Charlee is not unique in the results of her face-lift. Depending on how you looked before you saw the signs of age, you may see a change of twenty or twenty-five years, not ten. You can discuss with your surgeon what you want. Do you want eternal youth? Do you want to look as young as Cher, Goldie Hawn, or Jaclyn Smith? Maybe you can. Or you can be more conservative. It's up to you and your surgeon! Spend time with your doctor discussing what you have in mind. Be clear about the results you would like. Find out how close the surgeon can come to it. Then, if you want a face-lift, go for it!

FACE-LIFTS

Step by Step Through the Rhytidectomy, or Platysma Cervical Lift

There are several entire books written just on face-lifts. Don't hesitate to read them. They will give you a blow-by-blow. We'll give you all you need to know without the bells and whistles.

Before your face-lift.

First, review chapter 15 in this book, on preparing for surgery. If your doctor gives you instructions, remember that they are your Bible. You should be given them well in advance of the date when you are scheduled for surgery. If you don't understand why you are being asked to do or not do something, *ask!* But don't decide on your own to skip any instructions.

In the operating room.

A full face-lift can be performed in a physician's office, an outpatient surgical facility, or a hospital, depending upon the physician's and patient's evaluations and preferences. More and more, face-lifts are being done in a surgeon's fully equipped private operating facility, and you either go home after the operation, or recover overnight at the facility under professional supervision.

A face-lift can be done under general anesthesia, but usually it is done under local anesthesia and intravenous sedation. You may be given a Valium to take before you head to the surgeon's office, so be sure to have someone else drive you as well as pick you up afterward! When you get to the facility, you will probably be feeling a little stoned. This may, of course, be extremely pleasant and eliminate your pre-surgery jitters. Many doctors will give you a clonidine pill to lower your blood pressure before surgery. This not only reduces your bleeding, it helps prevent a hematoma (a pooling of blood under the skin) from forming after the surgery.

Some doctors intravenously administer antibiotics and steroids during the surgery. Some also give Zofran intravenously to prevent post-operative vomiting. Others will slip in a suppository toward the end of the procedure to prevent nausea after surgery. Both of those methods will alleviate much of your post-operative discomfort.

In the basic procedure, the surgeon works on one side of the face at a time. Incisions are made inside the hairline at the temple, running in front of the ear then around the earlobe and behind the ear, ending in the hair of the scalp. This incision may extend across the back of your head. You may also have a little incision under your chin, too, because this area is often liposuctioned and tightened up. The scar will look like one you might already have from childhood if you fell and hit your chin; no one will know it's from facial surgery.

HONEST TALK ABOUT SMOKING

You have a choice. If you are a smoker and can't stop, some doctors will not operate on you. Others may do a much more conservative procedure than if you were not smoking.

If you continue to smoke but still go ahead with your face-lift, you are at risk for more complications, particularly skin that dies (skin necrosis), leaving a large open wound, and hematomas (a collection of blood under the skin from bleeding).

If you are considering surgery, it is a good time to make the effort to stop smoking for good. If kicking the habit altogether is not an option for you, plan to stop at least a few days before your procedure. If you don't stop, you *must* tell your doctor. But no matter how addicted you are, you need to stop post-operatively for at least a few days (the longer the better, of course). So plan to tough it out. The nicotine patch is not an option (see page 246), but if you get desperate, go for the gum. It won't deliver a sustained dose like the patch, and you must limit yourself to a "survival" dose.

If you are having a rhinoplasty, a rare complication seen in heavy smokers is necrosis (dead tissue sloughing off) of the nasal tip. If this happens to you, you might need a skin graft, and certainly you will have an unsightly scar and/or a sunken area. While the complication is very uncommon, you are in control of whether it happens to you! Avoid the risk entirely by not smoking before or after the procedure (Benvenuti, 223).

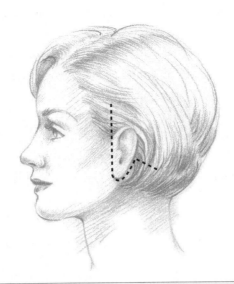

face-lift incisions

During the procedure, the skin is separated from the underlying tissue. The lax connective tissue and muscles of your face and neck are tightened up. Fat is removed or repositioned. The surgeon works like an artist, taking the signs of age from your face. The operation may take from three to five hours, depending on whether other procedures are done at the same time.

Special attention to your neck.

Unless you get a mini-lift, the surgeon using the PCL procedure will remove excess fat and tighten up the platysma muscle of your neck.

The platysma muscle once was a gill-opening muscle, used by our distant, fishy ancestors, and is the same muscle horses use to tighten their necks and chase flies away. This muscle is responsible for the bands on the neck, as well as the jowls that develop with age. Its division and tightening during a PCL does not impair facial expression in any way. As the platysma muscle is tightened, a sling is created that holds the face from the inside, placing little tension on the skin itself. You should end up with a beautiful contour from your chin to your neck, and a smooth, youthful neck. Some surgeons do "a great neck." It's worth really looking for one who excels at this. It's an "up" to be able to put on a beautiful necklace, even a "choker" or dog collar, maybe after years of avoiding them.

After the surgery is over, your face will be wrapped up in loose bandages that cover your entire head. Only a little bit of your face will show; think of an old-fashioned nun's habit with a wimple that hugs the face. You might even have two small cotton earplugs to prevent the oozing and drainage from the incision above your ears from creating a cleansing problem. The bandages are removed by your surgeon the day after surgery. You may have a drain under your incision as well. This, too, is removed painlessly when your bandages are taken off. If the bandage seems too tight or is otherwise uncomfortable, tell your doctor. *Do not take these bandages off on your own* (even if you are a nurse!). It is essential for these bandages to stay on for the first twenty-four hours.

Follow your surgeon's post-operative instructions to the letter. Study them. Have someone else study them. And don't cheat. It's only cheating yourself.

Special Tips on Getting Ready for Face-Lift Surgery

- If you dye your hair on a regular basis, get it done shortly before surgery. You can't get your roots done for four to six weeks afterward, so prepare as best you can. Also, see our tips below on purchasing clip-in hair extensions or falls.

- If you are limiting the number of people who you tell about your surgery, get your lies and stories ready. See our tips in chapter 16, "Secrets, Lies, or Full Disclosure," for ideas.

- Have clothes ready that do not have to be put on over your head. This includes nighties. *No T-Shirts unless they are V-Necked.*

> **WARNING**
>
> **Y**ou should not experience pain after a face-lift. Most girlfriends describe the sensation as "discomfort." If you experience pain in the face or if one side becomes hard or tense and is visibly larger than the other side, you must notify your doctor immediately.

Plan to have changes of clothing that button or zip up the front. Your head, my dear, should not be bumped, touched, squeezed, or rattled about. *Think* about it!

- Listen carefully. You may have difficulty talking. You won't want to move your face much. You may not be able to talk immediately after surgery. Take our advice: don't see people—even family. Let people see you *after* you are looking good—otherwise you are going to be in for some grief from their comments. You will look worse than you feel. In fact, you will probably feel great and look awful. Your family may go nuts on you. Spare them. In a week you'll look pretty darn good. In two weeks, you'll look great. Don't see people until then. *Trust* us!

- Plan to limit phone calls. . . . Let's be even stronger about that: Don't *have* phone calls. Don't accept them. Don't make them. Have someone else call relatives and friends to tell them that you are doing fine and that you will talk to them in a few days. Why? You will have difficulty holding a phone to your ear or moving your face to talk. If you must use the phone, use a speakerphone.

Tips on Going Out After Surgery

- Makeup can be applied a few days after the stitches are removed. For example, if your stitches are removed on day ten you can apply makeup on day fourteen, or about two weeks after surgery. Use a hypoallergenic camouflaging makeup (see the listing of brands on page 197).

- Sunblock of SPF 15 or above should be used on all incisions for a minimum of four to six months after the surgery to prevent hyperpigmentation, or darkening of the skin.

- Do not wear *anything* you need to put on over your head—sweaters, turtlenecks, shirts, or blouses—for *three weeks* after the surgery. Here's what happened to girlfriend Raquel:

I was feeling really good after getting my stitches out, so my sister-in-law and I left the doctor's office and headed for the mall. An hour later I'm in a dressing room trying on a turtleneck, and as I pulled it back over my head to take it off, it caught my earlobe. The turtleneck nearly tore my entire ear off my head. It opened up the whole incision, and I'm standing there with my ear loose, the blood running, and me screaming. My sister-in-law stayed calm and got a towel from a salesgirl. We ended up rushing back to my plastic surgeon's office with me holding the towel to my ear. What a mess. I was sure I tore my ear right off. Fortunately, it wasn't nearly that bad, but I was scared! So *don't* pull anything tight on or off over your head until you are good and healed!

- Do not wearing earrings for *six weeks!* Girlfriends, listen carefully. You can rip your earlobe off all too easily if you wear earrings after a face-lift.

  Here's the real deal: Your ear is used to camouflage the incisions of your surgery. There is tension on these incisions, as if you took three pieces of material and sewed them so every piece touched the other. The place where all three pieces join is critical and very stressed. If you catch your earring on anything—remember, your earlobe is numb—you can do tremendous damage without knowing it. Don't cheat. Don't even think about cheating. *Don't wear earrings for six weeks!*

- Do not chew gum for two weeks. The motion of your jaw can place tension on the incision behind the ear and disturb the healing process in this area. If you need to avoid smoking, nicotine gum takes very little chewing before it is "parked" next to your cheek to release its dose. Just use sparingly and chew gently.

You will not see the results of your face-lift until at least three months have passed, and it is not until after six months have passed that you will see the full benefits. You will continue to see subtle changes for up to a year following your surgery (May, 193).

What to Expect Medically After Your Surgery

- A slight amount of drainage from the stitchline for the first few days after the bandage is removed. You may *gently* wash the crusts that form with *mild* soap and *cool* or *warm* water.

- Mild discomfort or a slight headache. You should *not* experience pain.

- A feeling of tightness. This is especially noticeable in the lower face and neck.

- Bruising is normal after this procedure. The bruises usually fade completely in about three weeks.

- Swelling is normal after this procedure—at its worst the first week after surgery. During the second week, the swelling begins to subside but some fullness persists. The bonus to this is you won't have a line or wrinkle on your face, and girlfriends lament that some do come back when the swelling subsides. So expect some return of lines. By the end of the month, 75 percent of the swelling is usually gone, but the

HAIR LOSS—WHAT TO DO

Girlfriends, don't get hysterical when you see your hair going down the drain the first time you wash your hair after a face-lift or a brow-lift. You will lose a lot. This is a big problem with fine-haired blondes, especially. Your hair *will* grow back—but it takes months. What to do? Get clip-in hair extensions or "falls." Ask your beautician what she or he recommends, too. Some girlfriends had expensive hair-weaves after their incisions healed. There are some new processes for hair extensions on the market, too. They are expensive, but depending on how much hair you are missing, you will feel better if you plan ahead for a temporary replacement.

swelling does not completely resolve itself until three to four months after surgery.

- Flaking and peeling skin. Edema, or swelling, will cause the top layer of your skin to eventually slough off—in other words it will get all flaky and peel. This is not a medical problem, but girlfriends complain about it a lot because it really makes your makeup look awful. It goes away in a day or two.

- Numbness. You may be completely numb on the sides of your face extending to your cheek area. The feeling will slowly return, although some areas may remain less sensitive than before surgery.

- There will be scars, but they should be inconspicuous. The ones in front of your ears should disappear completely or nearly so. Behind the ear you may be left with a noticeable scar, but it can easily be covered by your hair. The incisions across the back of your head will be hidden completely by your hair.

- Temporary hair loss. You might want to get a few "falls" or clip-in hairpieces to give the appearance of fullness until your hair grows back.

STRAIGHT TALK ABOUT COMPLICATIONS

A face-lift is one of the safest procedures. Two minor aftereffects are common:

1. Numbness—this eventually goes away when the nerves heal, although some areas may remain desensitized.

2. Bumps or lumps—these raised areas may appear on cheeks during the first weeks of healing. Regular massaging of the area or use of steroid creams will help them disappear. Eventually, they do go away.

WHEN TO CALL YOUR DOCTOR

- If you are nauseous the night after surgery and are not staying overnight at a medical facility. (You do not want to vomit. A suppository can stop your nausea.)

- If you experience sudden or prolonged pain.

- If an area of your face or neck begins to swell out of proportion to the rest of your face, especially in the first two to three days after surgery, or on the eighth to tenth days.

- If the area around the incision exudes pus or looks infected.

- If the area around the incision begins to separate and open.

LATE-BLEEDING WARNING

A rare but serious hematoma, caused by bleeding from the superficial temporal artery (located on the right side of the face), seems to sometimes occur, between eight and ten days after the face-lift. Not associated with infection, bleeding from the superficial temporal vessels is probably caused by a rise in blood pressure from activities such as lifting, bending over and working in the garden, sports and jogging—or from taking aspirin or vitamin E. Girlfriends, please note that one of the most common causes of late bleeding is vigorous intercourse (Grazer, 767). Patients sometimes describe hearing a "pop." If this happens to you, apply pressure in front of and above the ear, call 911, and contact your surgeon at once (Jones, 577).

Other complications do happen, but they are relatively rare. They nearly always can be resolved with your doctor's help. Here is an overview:

- A hematoma is the most common complication following a face-lift. The reported incidence of hematoma has ranged from 0.3 to 8.1 percent, but is increasing due to the habitual use of vitamin E. Large, expanding hematomas can result in partial skin loss, an increased incidence of infection, skin hyperpigmentation, persistent facial swelling, numbness, and a prolonged convalescence (Rees, 1185). Hematomas may be caused by a rise in blood pressure, taking aspirin products, or long-term ingestion of vitamin E (see page 247). Most hematomas occur within one to fifteen hours after surgery, or around forty-eight hours after surgery. However, hematomas pose a danger for the first two weeks. A small number (2 percent) of hematomas require draining by your doctor.

- Other complications are inflammation (5 percent); crusting of suture lines (3.25 percent); raised scars, behind ear (1.5 percent); hair loss, temples (1.25 percent)—if this is severe, single-hair grafts, or transplants, may be used to correct it (Kaye et al, panel discussion); and an adhesion behind the earlobe (1 percent).

- Very rare complications, less than 1 percent, include persistent pain (usually at the temple); stitch abscesses; generalized bruising; herpes of lips; compromised circulation; seroma (fluid under the skin); dilated veins of cheeks; raised scars requiring revision; temporary parotid fistula (a depression near the ear); tissue necrosis; hyperpigmentation; acne eruption; motor nerve loss (most injuries are due to bruising or stretching of the nerves, and the problem usually resolves in three to six months, even in six weeks, sometimes) (panel, 49); cyst development (Hamilton, 207); or "shotgun" neck deformity, when too much fat is removed from under the chin.

Again, girlfriends, complications are uncommon, but if they do happen, almost none of them are permanent. Be patient and work with your doctor on resolving them.

THE BIG QUESTION: HOW LONG DOES A FACE-LIFT LAST?

It's a myth that a face-lift "falls." It doesn't. Bluntly put, a face-lift does not last forever and it cannot "stop the clock." Time marches on. You will continue to age at the same rate you did before your lift. However, you will always look better and more youthful than you would have if you never had one. Research also shows that you will have more skin elasticity compared with those in the same age group who have never had surgery (Guyuron, 1284).

Now, to be direct about what you really want to know: Here's the truth about face-lifts, straight from the shoulder:

NO MORE HIGH COLLARS AND TURTLENECKS

Girlfriends, be prepared to buy some new clothes after your face-lift heals. Your neck and jawline are going to look terrific, so show them off! Get ready to splurge on

- Plunging necklines
- Scoop necks
- Flattering V-necks
- Short necklaces: dog collars, chokers, rigid gold wires, and short chains
- Long earrings to dangle down to your jawline, drawing the eyes to your new look

And while bunched turtlenecks and scarves are lovely, you don't *need* to wear them to hide anything. Now you have freedom of choice!

And, oh yes . . . If you only have a single piercing of your ears, it's time to add another, and another. Because, lady, you look fabulous.

- A good neck job should last ten years.

- A good face-lift should last five years.

- You will see laxity in the midface after about three years.

However, most girlfriends wait an average of 8.48 years (1- to 16-year spread) before having a second lift (Guyuron, 1281). *But,* there are several "maintenance" procedures you can do to make your lift look better longer.

- Botox! This "quick fix" eliminates frown lines between the eyes or on the forehead, and other dynamic wrinkles. Injected into the site of the wrinkle, the first treatment will wear off in a few months or less. The second may last up to a year. For some women, the third treatment is almost permanent. (See more about Botox on pages 215–17.)

- AlloDerm implants. These implants are surgically placed through small incisions. They can plump up lips, nasolabial folds, and a cleft between the eyes. (See more about Allo-Derm on page 219.)

- Cheek implants. They will help fill out a lax midface and give back definition. (See more about cheek implants on pages 163–65.)

- Laser resurfacing. Laser can eliminate wrinkles and leave your skin beautiful . . . if you don't have any complications. Pros and cons are discussed in depth on pages 186–95.

- Brow-lift. If this procedure wasn't part of your original face-lift; doing it a few years later can renew and refresh your look. Check out the details on pages 159–61.

- Blepharoplasty. Although the lower lids are usually done along with your face-lift, your upper lids may not be. Review the particulars on this surgery on pages 150–59.

- Mini face-lift, or endoscopic lift. A mini-lift is really a second lift without the neck, but it is less costly and does a terrific job.

The difficulty? Not every plastic surgeon does them, or can do them well.

- Glycolic peels, mini-dermabrasion, Retin-A, and alpha-hydroxy creams. All of these should be part of your regular skin-care program. You can find the details in section 4, "Getting the Wrinkles Out."

The trade-offs of a face-lift.

Despite all the wonderful benefits of a good face-lift, there are some negatives. First, you will have scars—not big, not bad, but they are there.

You will have some hair loss. Most hair lost at the time of surgery grows back, and any permanent loss is usually not noticeable. You may lose some of your sideburns, especially with second or more surgeries (Kaye, 198).

Outside of the scars and hair loss, girlfriends, the benefits far outweigh any losses. A face-lift is the closest thing to true rejuvenation we have.

A NEW 'DO FOR THE NEW YOU

You may want to change your hairstyle after surgery, and not just because of temporary hair loss. Until the incisions in front of the ears fade, you will want a hairstyle that covers this area. Also, because larger scars are usually left visible behind the ears, you might think twice about pulling long hair tightly back into a ponytail, French braid, or twist. Sometimes this anterior scar can be very noticeable. Charlee once had a date ask what the scar was. Hmm, was she detecting a knowing sneer in the question? Since her date wasn't someone she felt like "sharing" her face-lift experience with (when it comes to men, some don't need to know—ever), she answered, very matter-of-factly, "I had mastoid surgery when I was a child." The guy let the subject drop and didn't ask what "mastoid surgery" was, but in case you decide to use this white lie and want to be prepared: Mastoiditis is an inflammation of the mastoid, a bone behind the ear. In mastoid surgery, or a mastoidectomy, part or all of the bone is removed. If anyone wants to know more than that—hell, you were only six and you don't remember much about it. If you need to, answer the question with a question and ask the nosy fellow if he has prostate trouble, after all most men of a certain age do. *Meow.*

8

OTHER FACIAL PROCEDURES

Want fabulous cheekbones? A little less chin? A smooth forehead again? Often a subtle change that affects the balance of a woman's face can transform her from "attractive" to "drop-dead gorgeous." These lesser-known procedures are called ancillary ("associated") procedures. Many of them are commonly performed at the same time as a face-lift. After all, if you're getting nipped and tucked, why not end up with a model's angular bones? No one but your surgeon will know they're plastic. Other than increasing the time of the surgery and the recovery period, these procedures don't increase the risk. Also, by combining procedures into one operation, you can save on the anesthesia and facility fees, and that may reduce costs. But surgery on your eyes, a brow-lift, chin work, cheek implants, nose jobs, and other facial surgeries can also be done alone, before or after your face-lift, as conditions and years dictate.

The most common ancillary procedures affect the eyes: a blepharoplasty of either your upper and lower lids or both, and a forehead/brow-lift. Younger women in their late twenties and thirties are having blepharoplasty surgery and successfully maintaining a very refreshed, youthful look. But even older women in their seventies can get great results. In fact, nearly two hundred thousand women had blepharoplasties in 1998 (American Society for Aesthetic Plastic Surgery).

THE EYES HAVE IT

Blepharoplasty of the Lower Lids

Girlfriends, how long have you been applying concealer to hide the bags under your eyes? All they do is get worse as the years roll by. Some girlfriends have inherited pouches, others just get crepey and puffy, and others get "basset-hound eyes," as their eyes droop and the whites begin to show. The biggest effect is that you not only look older, but you look *tired*. This, girlfriends, can have a negative effect on your work life. At that point, blepharoplasty is not a matter of vanity; it is a matter of economics.

Take Jeannie. She is a sales rep for a major pharmaceutical company. When she was passed over for a promotion to a regional manager, she thought, *Aha, it's because I'm a woman.* She put in for a transfer to another office, fuming, wondering if she should bring a discrimination suit, and wondering what to do.

She decided to work twice as hard. Jeannie took off in her new office, wowing everyone. Her figures were good. Her work impressive. Then one day her boss asked her if she'd been working too hard; she looked tired—did she want some time off?

Jeannie was taken aback. She *wasn't* tired.

A couple of weeks later, the "tired look" was brought to her attention again. "You must have had some weekend," a young, twenty-something sales rep said one Monday morning. He had come in straight from his morning workout at the gym. His hair was still wet from his shower. He looked like he could run a marathon without getting winded. Jeannie gave him a suspicious look. She was only thirty-five—not that old. She still could be having wild weekends.

"Not really," she said. "Why do you think so?"

"Well, you look beat! Wiped out, you know?"

The Arctic doesn't have frost deeper than Jeannie's icy reply. But when she was alone in her office, she took out her compact and looked at herself. Fluorescent lights aren't flattering. She saw a tired, haggard face. She told us,

> I had to face facts. I *did* look tired. I had bags under my eyes and deep wrinkles on my cheekbones. I wasn't even forty and I looked middle-aged. I really felt my job security was on the line. After a moment of panic, I calmed down and decided to do something about it. My mother had gotten eyelid surgery when she was in her sixties. Okay, I figured. I could do it. So I called her doctor and made an appointment.
>
> What was so funny, nobody at work knew about my surgery—or even guessed. I took two weeks' vacation and told people I was going to Cancún. All anybody said when I went back to work was that I looked great.
>
> I looked right at the young sales rep and said, "Oh, I had a wild time."
>
> I not only got a big promotion six months later, but get this: That kid asked me out!

Fortunately, as Jeannie found out, getting just the lower eyelid rejuvenated is a wonderfully easy procedure that is virtually undetectable after it heals. An incision is made along the line of the lower lashes, or directly below the pink part, or conjunctiva. If you have a large pouch under your eye, the fat may be removed. However, newer thinking in facial surgery emphasizes *moving* the fat when possible instead of removing it. Fat sustains and holds up your skin.

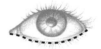

lower blepharoplasty

The wrinkled and crepelike skin under your eye is pulled up and cut off. Then the incision is closed with tiny sutures and covered with flesh-colored Band-Aids or Steri-Strips™. The doctor will remove these in a few days. When the incision completely heals, it is impossible, or nearly impossible, to see any scars. The results are spectacular.

Upper lids too?

Not seeing your eyeshadow anymore is only part of the problem when you gets "hoods" instead of lids. The skin on your upper lids, right up to your eyebrow, can droop so badly it will obscure your peripheral vision. Want to know what can be good about that? Your health insurance *may* help pay for an upper blepharoplasty, particularly if you are sixty or above, if your ophthalmologist recommends it, and if you pass a "peripheral field study." Find more details in chapter 14, "Finding the Money."

For an upper blepharoplasty, an incision is made in the fold of the lid, and excess fat and/or skin is removed. Again, very tiny stitches close the incision.

Both upper and lower eyelid surgery can be done in the doctor's office with local anesthesia only or with intravenous sedation and local anesthesia. In either case, the patient is placed in a total state of relaxation during the procedure and goes home shortly afterward. Because sedative drugs are used during the procedure, you will need someone to drive you home. You will also have blurry vision from the ointment in your eyes. Your

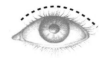

upper blepharoplasty

vision is *always* compromised right after surgery. *You will not be able to drive.* Take a cab if you have to, but plan on getting home *without driving.*

Girlfriends' Tips to Get Ready for Eye Surgery

- Get yourself a gorgeous new pair of sunglasses.

- Go out and get all new eye makeup. This is fun—and serious business. Makeup becomes heavily contaminated with germs. Start fresh when you finally get the okay to resume use after surgery.

- If you aren't telling people about your surgery, prepare your story about how you got your bruises (see our tips in chapter 16, "Secrets, Lies, or Full Disclosure"). This operation is one *no one needs to know about!* You will look rested; you will look younger—but most people will not realize why. If you don't want to tell, don't. Once your bruises and incisions heal, no one will ever know if you don't tell them.

RECOVERY TIME FOR A BLEPHAROPLASTY

It takes about two to three weeks to recover fully from this surgery, but by three to four days after the procedure, you can usually travel outside. You can drive only when you no longer need to put ointment in your eyes. Most girlfriends return to work between seven and ten days after surgery. Some working women go back to work as early as four days, while others may require a full three weeks for all the bruising to disappear.

You can apply makeup on the incision site within two to four days *after your stitches are removed.* You can always put makeup on other parts of your face. If you have a lower blepharoplasty, you certainly can wear eyeliner and shadow on the upper lids. Watch the mascara, however, as it can smudge.

Most of the stitches used in the eyelids are dissolvable, but a few will need removal. Two to three days after having a blepharoplasty, the patient returns to the doctor's office, at which time sutures that have been secured by Steri-Strips are removed. Additional flesh-colored Steri-Strips may be applied after the skin is cleansed gently with a degreaser. These tapes will stay in place until the one-week post-operative visit, at which time most tapes are removed and their use is discontinued.

Girlfriend Anne cautions not to go back to work too soon.

I had my lower lids done on a Friday. I kept ice on my eyes and followed instructions to the letter. I didn't even have any bruising—until I went back to work on Monday. While I was working at my desk, I unconsciously kept my face angled slightly down. Before I knew it, my eyes puffed up enormously and that's when I bruised. If I stayed out of work just an extra day or two, I would have recovered much faster. Instead, I "rushed" going back to work and slowed up my healing. My advice: Take as much time off as you can.

Your surgeon will give you post-operative instructions. *Don't do anything on your own . . . and don't do anything simply because that's what a friend did.*

Girlfriends' Tips for Your Recovery

- Wear those new dark glasses both inside and outside. They will camouflage your surgery, rest the eyes, prevent strain, and add to your overall comfort.

- Wear a sunblock of SPF 15 or more around your eyes until all bruising is gone—*and on all incision sites for a minimum of four to six months after surgery.* The sun interferes with healing and may cause excessive redness and itching. It can also cause hyper-pigmentation (darker skin), which will take longer to fade.

- Makeup can be applied two to four days *after* the eyelid sutures are removed (see discussion above). Hypoallergenic paramedical makeup products (see list on page 197) are usually well-tolerated and effective as cover-ups.

What to Expect Medically After Eyelid Surgery

- A small amount of bloody drainage for three to five days after the surgery.

- Crust or dried blood around the incisions. You may gently wash or cleanse this with plain, cool water or half-strength hydrogen peroxide. Blot rather than rub. Don't use so much it runs into your eyes. Use "no tears" baby shampoo if you would like to use a little soap.

- Blurry vision for a few days due to seepage of ointment into the eyes themselves.

- Burning or itchiness in the eyes or eyelids. This can be treated by the nightly application of Celluvisc, Lacri-Lube, or some other comparable eye lubricant.

- Bruising and swelling. Diligent application of ice packs, oral vitamin C, arnica montana, and vitamin K cream will speed healing. Normally, bruising is completely resolved by three weeks.

- Mild discomfort. You should *not* experience pain after this procedure.

- Your eyes may not close completely for one to two weeks after the surgery. They may feel tight at first, but this feeling goes away when the stitches are removed. Once the stitches are out, you will begin eye exercises to improve the ability of the eyes to close. These exercises involve squinting your eyelids together for ten rapid repetitions at least three times a day per day for one to two weeks.

- Numbness. Small nerves to the skin may be interrupted during surgery. Your eyelids may feel numb or have less than full feeling for a period anywhere from several weeks to months. This is more a nuisance than a medical problem. Occasionally, some diminished sensitivity may last indefinitely.

- Redness around the eyes and incision sites. This will fade in three to four months. You can cover it up with makeup after the sutures are removed.

- Scars. All scars tend to fade with time and eventually look like thin, fine white lines . . . or are completely invisible. However, the final width, height, color, and appearance cannot be predicted before surgery. The final outcome depends on a variety of factors including genetics, individual skin chemistry, nutrition, smoking, post-operative care, and one's overall healing capacity.

Expect to see gradual improvement in the appearance of your eyes for three to six months. As healing continues, the final result will emerge. The results of this surgery can be spectacular, but you must be patient during the healing phase.

Rosemary C. says,

Before my upper blepharoplasty, I already had had a face-lift and my nose fixed. I felt like a veteran. So I didn't read the doctor's instructions. After all, I'd been through this before. I woke up in the wee hours with excruciating pain in my eyes. I thought I was having some horrible complication. Of course, I became panicky and called the doctor in the middle of the night. What was the problem? My eyes, still unable to completely close, had gotten dry—because I had neglected to put the prescribed drops in my eyes before I went to bed. My advice is to read *all* of the instructions, even if you've had surgery before. Nobody knows it all.

COMPLICATIONS

Medical complications are rare after a blepharoplasty, but here are a few potential problems.

- Infection is a possibility, but it is unlikely because you will probably receive antibiotics for five days after surgery.

- There is a remote possibility that some blood or serum may collect under the skin (hematoma or seroma). If this occurs, it can usually be readily evacuated in the doctor's office, although occasionally, a patient may require a return to the operating room for treatment. With appropriate treatment, your results will not be affected.

- Pain can also be a symptom of an abrasion of the cornea, which may occur if you accidentally rub your eye.

- Lost stitch. Occasionally, a stitch can come out, which is easily fixed.

- Tearing, dry eyes, and photosensitivity (sensitivity to light) are also possible complications.

But, more common than the medical complications above, are less-than-great results, including the following.

WHEN TO CALL YOUR DOCTOR

- If there is excessive bleeding or swelling.

- If you experience pain in the eyes or if one side becomes hard or tense and is visibly larger than the other side.

- If blurry vision persists after the prescribed ointment has been discontinued or if visual acuity (sharpness of vision) diminishes for any reason.

- Too much off the upper lids. This can cause corneal exposure, which can result in sensitivity to light, tearing, dry eyes, and pain (Hurwitz, 149–50).

- Too much off the lower lids. The eyelid may retract from the globe and expose the sclera (the white of the eye) below the pupil and the conjunctiva (the pink shelf).

- Eyes that lack symmetry, or appear narrower, with an unnatural appearance and stare. Some women complain of "asymmetrical eyes" after blepharoplasty; in other words, they complain that their two eyes are different. Girlfriends, your two eyes *are* different. Whatever you have two of on your body—hands, feet, ears, eyebrows, breasts—*are* different. The two sides of your entire body, and the two sides of your face, are different. When you take a photo, you have a "good side" and a "bad side." Marilyn Monroe, for instance, tried to avoid having a photo taken of her left side.

  Try this test. Take a piece of cardboard, or anything stiff, and center it vertically down your face. Look at one side at a time. You will see two very different "looks." After surgery you will be looking closely at your eyes. They will not be exactly the same because they weren't the same before the operation. Asymmetry is only a problem if it is extreme. Some unevenness is normal!

Remember, any problems usually resolve in time and with your doctor's help. However, your best guarantee against unfavorable results from a blepharoplasty is to choose your doctor wisely. Angie adds,

My ophthalmologist is the doctor who recommended I have a blepharoplasty because my upper eyelids were drooping so badly they were hampering my ability to see, especially when I drove. He said insurance would cover the procedure, and he could do it. *Oh no!* I thought. *If anyone is going to cut my face, I'm going to a plastic surgeon who does this operation all the time and is concerned with how I look . . . not just how I'm able to see.*

The Best News

The results of this surgery should last forever. A blepharoplasty is usually a once-in-a-lifetime operation. The vast majority of patients who have this surgery will not need any additional eyelid rejuvenation for as long as they live.

But wait a minute. . . . With the upper lids, you have a choice. Sometimes a brow-lift is a better idea, so read about that, too, before you decide.

THE BROW- AND FOREHEAD-LIFT

Brow-lifts have been done by surgeons for a long time; in fact, the first plastic-surgery textbook, published in 1919, discusses them. The basic "bicoronal" brow-lift has been used since 1962 (Byrd, 928). Usually done in an office facility, using local anesthetic and intravenous sedation, this type of forehead- and brow-lift requires an incision made across the top of the head from the front of one ear to the front of the other ear. The incision may be made deep within the frontal hairline to hide the resulting scar.

With a traditional lift, the forehead and brows are elevated, and excess skin is removed. The nerves to the muscles that cause the "frown" or cleft between your eyes are also cut. This keeps you from being able to frown. Oddly enough, these nerves will regenerate in 50 percent of patients, and the frown returns. (If that happens, try Botox; see pages 215–17.) If you have a long-standing indentation or cleft, it can be filled at this time with an AlloDerm implant. The ridges in your brow will disappear or be diminished;

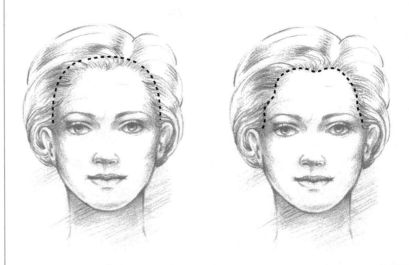

brow-lift incision

however, some will return in time. Because your eyebrows are lifted, the excess skin on your upper eyelids is stretched, and some, or even most, of the drooping is eliminated.

Girlfriends, you should realize that your brows will always be higher after this surgery. This can result in a permanent look of "surprise." However, for most women, the results are very positive, or even spectacular.

Bruising from this surgery is moderate to minimal, and the swelling lasts a few weeks. You will experience some hair loss along the incision line, so you might want to use "falls" or clip-in hair until your hair grows back, to restore a look of fullness. The biggest complaint after a brow-lift is the feeling of numbness at the top of your head. It probably *won't* go away.

Girlfriends can follow the tips for face-lift post-op care, although you will find this operation is much less traumatic. However, you still have to be careful and thoughtful, no matter how good you feel. One girlfriend had this experience:

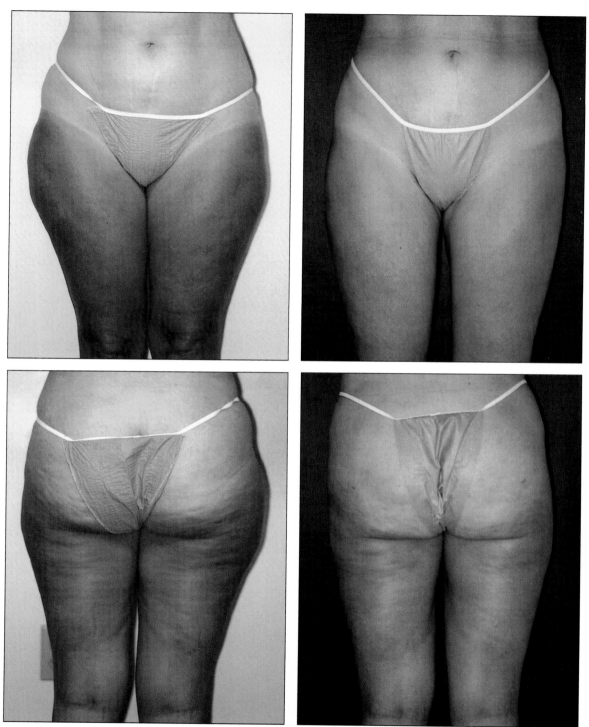

Great liposuction results on typical thunder thighs. Girlfriends, the sad truth is that all the exercise in the world can't get rid of saddle bags, but liposuction can.

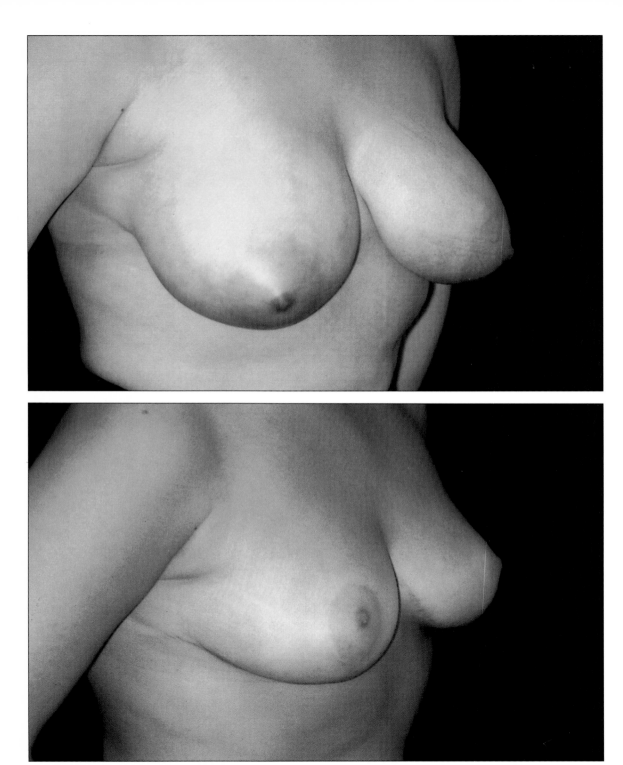

This girlfriend looks fabulous after her breast reduction surgery. Notice that there is scarring, but it's subtle.

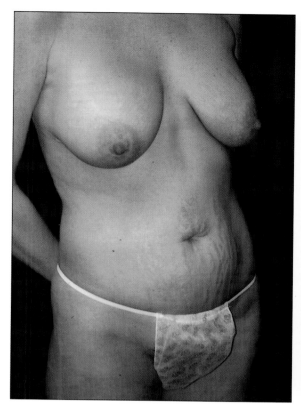
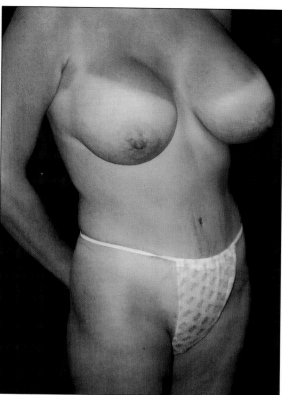

Pregnancy did a number on this girlfriend, but, with the exception of some remaining stretch marks, her breast augmentation and tummy tuck put everything back in its rightful place.

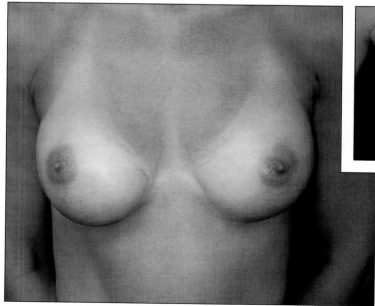
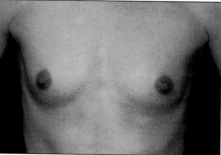

Catherine went from flat to fabulous. This is a beautiful breast augmentation.

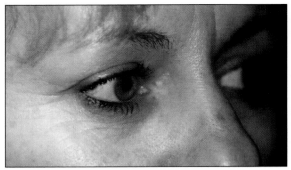
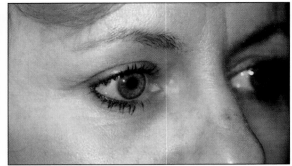

Laser resurfacing for crow's feet. The lines around the corner of the eyes are significantly less noticeable. Is it worth the down time and risk? This girlfriend says "yes!"

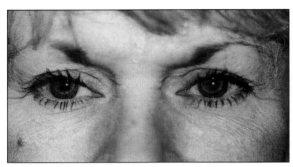
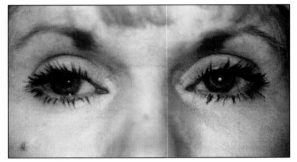

Upper and lower eyelid lift. Now you see those awful pouches, now you don't. And as an added bonus, there are no visible scars.

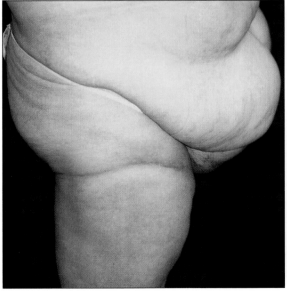
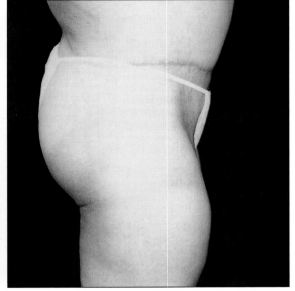

This girlfriend had multiple procedures performed: radical fat and skin reduction surgery, and a tummy tuck. Shocking? You bet. Don't think this lady hadn't tried to lose weight. Surgery gave her a new lease on life.

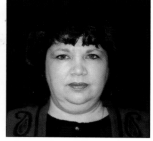

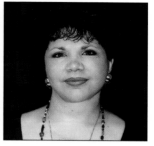

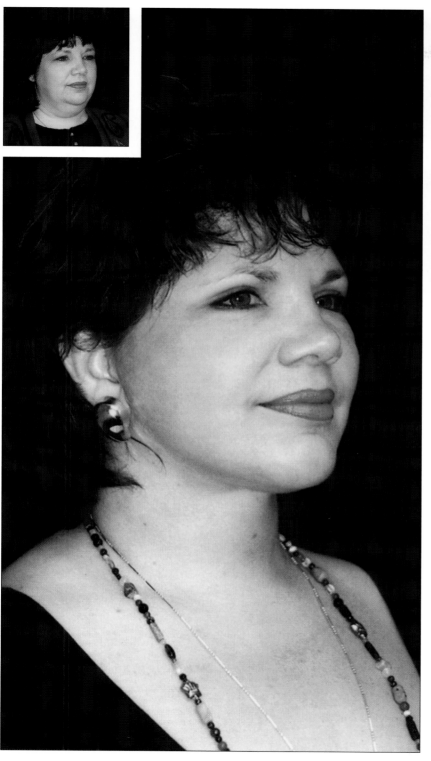

Mother and daughter? No! This is the same girlfriend after a face-lift and upper and lower lid surgery. You can imagine how her life must have changed.

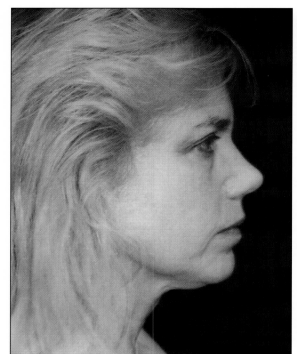
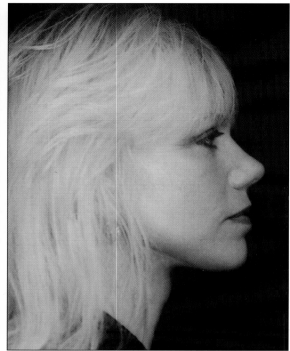

Here's Charlee before and after her face-lift and lower eyelid surgeries. Dr. Collini turned the clock back, way back.

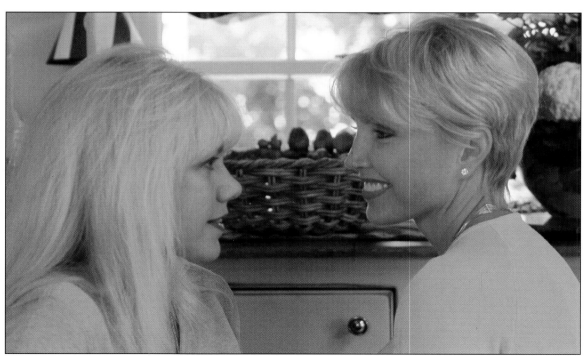

Charlee and Susan, ageless girlfriends forever.

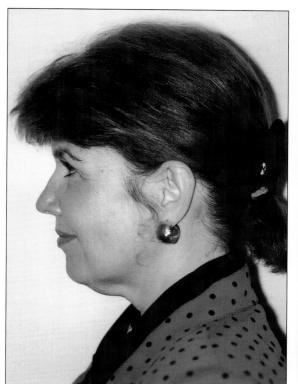
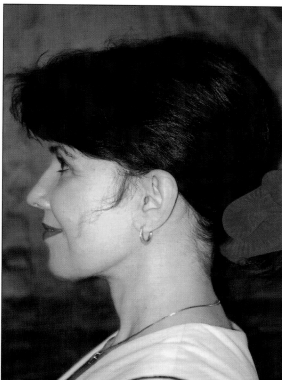

This is our favorite face-lift and eyelid surgery result. Isn't this one like a dream come true? This woman is oh, so young again.

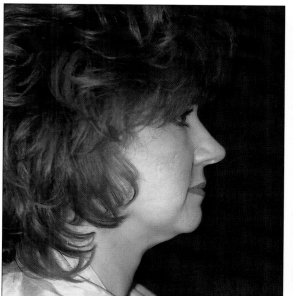
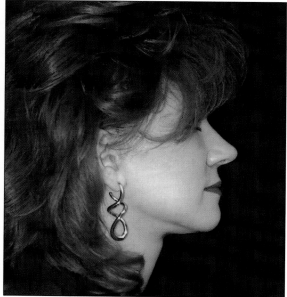

A nice, classic face-lift. Notice the neck and the loss of what, twenty years?

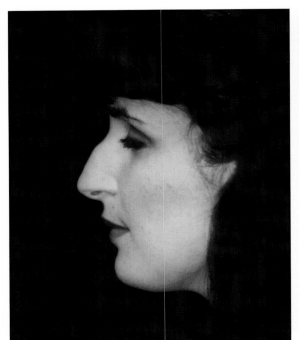 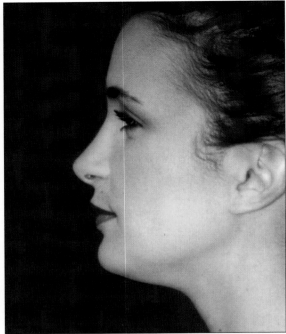

After Cindy's rhinoplasty, she sobbed when she saw her perfect "little" nose instead of the classic Roman nose that dominated her delicate face for thirty years. She looks exquisite.

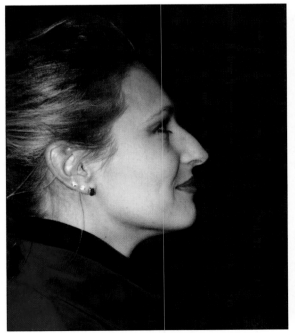 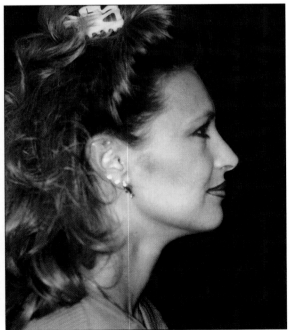

This is a rhinoplasty case with great results. Not only is the bump gone, but the nose is slightly shortened as well. Do you think a nose job also makes a person look younger? We do!

I had gotten my stitches out and was finally able to shampoo my hair myself. You know me, always rushing. Well, I was going back to work the next morning, and as usual I was running late. My girlfriend picked me up and I didn't have time to blow-dry. When I got in the car, my hair—which is quite short—was still wet. It was hot out, and as I was getting chilled from the air-conditioning, I rolled down the window and stuck my head out to "air-dry." It worked great, until I pulled my head back into the car and miscalculated the height of the window. I hit my head with a glancing blow on the car-door rim, and completely opened up the top of my head. The blood was gushing down my face while my girlfriend raced me to the emergency room where they called my plastic surgeon. Boy, did I feel dumb explaining how I did it!

A brow-lift is an alternative to a blepharoplasty to correct drooping upper eyelids, and it will address a wrinkled forehead, drooping brows, and frown lines. It also leaves you the option to get a blepharoplasty farther along in life as the aging process continues.

The trade-offs.

To get the benefits of a brow-lift you must expect scars, numbness of the scalp, higher eyebrows, and the eventual return of dynamic wrinkles in the forehead or even between the eyes.

THE PROBLEM OF NASOLABIAL FOLDS

Remember Denise's "Grand Canyons" (see pages 125–27)? The nasolabial folds that extend from the nose to the corners of the mouth are tough to eliminate, and women hate them! Ivana Trump, whose face looks great otherwise, is plagued with "Grand Canyons," too. A face-lift may lessen the nasolabial folds' appearance, but maybe not as much as you would like. Worse, these grooves and pouches may return (sometimes as quickly as two weeks!) after a face-lift if your plastic surgeon doesn't take special care to address them (Millard, 45). Several methods have been tried and proven to remove the nasolabial fold, and an experienced plastic surgeon can make a dramatic improvement in their appearance. If nasolabial folds are a distressing problem for you, discuss the options with your surgeon. Ask to see pictures of other cases he or she has corrected.

Here are some possible approaches you might consider after a face-lift that didn't "cure" them or before you are ready for a lift.

- Liposuction. It reduces the fat but leaves the slack skin of the nasolabial folds even more slack. It is most effective in younger patients with good skin elasticity (Millard, 37). But liposuction in the face is *very* controversial, because it can leave unevenness or streaks. In general, we don't recommend it.

- Buccal fat-pad removal and cheek implants. Buccal fat pads are the fat that causes "chipmunk cheeks." It looks like a golfball of fat when easily removed through an incision inside the mouth on the inner cheek. The incision is closed with absorbable stitches. A cheek implant (see pages 163–65) further pulls the remaining lax skin up. Denise had this procedure done (along with AlloDerm implants), and she said that although she had swelling for over a week, there was no pain and no problem eating.

- Cutting them out (direct excision of the folds). Cutting out the area works . . . but leaves cheek scars. They may not be very noticeable, but aren't desirable. This procedure is out of favor.

- Fat or collagen injections (see pages 217–19). You can fill up the folds with collagen or your own fat, but the results aren't permanent. Your body reabsorbs the collagen or fat, but some fat may remain and improve the folds' appearance.

- AlloDerm implants can be inserted up into the folds through incisions in the mouth, or down from incisions made below the eyes. The AlloDerm implant is long-lasting and really helps. Girlfriend Rosemary C., however, had one of her implants shift its position, and she had to go back for another procedure to correct it.

A combination of cheek implants, buccal fat-pad removal, and AlloDerm has given the best results we've seen. Discuss the situation long and carefully with your surgeon before you make a final decision on what to do.

THE CLASSY LOOK OF CHEEK IMPLANTS

Put a dab of highlighter on the cheeks below the outside corners of your eyes. Take your favorite color blush and bring it down diagonally, beneath your actual cheekbones. Your goal is to create the illusion of high cheekbones—and until recently, if you weren't born with them, makeup was your only option.

Now, "malar augmentation," or cheek implants, can give women the high cheekbones they desire. Girlfriends with long, narrow faces, or with very round faces and flat cheeks, get the best

---

HEAR, HEAR! DON'T FORGET YOUR EARLOBES

First women—and men—had one hole per ear lobe for a pierced earring. Now, *two* holes are considered conservative. We love to adorn our ears; in fact, dangling earrings that move with your body are said to increase the impression of femininity. More and more, we are drawing attention to our ears, yet one facial feature that everyone notices but few people talk about is the earlobe. First of all, earlobes tend to get longer as you get older. An option during your face-lift surgery (or anytime) is to have your earlobes shortened! Second, an attached earlobe may be less attractive than a detached one. Yes, your surgeon can detach it, and with some techniques, it won't even leave a scar (panel, 49).

results from these implants. Cheek implants will also benefit women with asymmetries or congenital defects. The procedure can be done at the same time as a face-lift or a surgery of the eyes (blepharoplasty), or it can be done on its own. The surgery is frequently performed in the doctor's facility under local anesthesia and intravenous sedation.

Cheek implants come in different sizes, and your surgeon will carefully measure your face to determine size and placement. To place the implant, an incision is made either in the mouth, or immediately below the lower eyelids. In the mouth, the most frequent route, the incision is made between the upper gums and the cheek. The soft tissue is lifted, creating a pocket over the cheekbone. The implant, which is triangular in shape, is then inserted. Tiny sutures are used to close the incisions. And, for about three days, little weights are fastened to the implants on *the outside of your cheeks* with a stitch through your skin! This sounds awful, looks strange, but doesn't hurt. Its purpose is to keep the implant in place while your face heals.

Sutures are removed within a week; pain should be minimal. Your face will be swollen in the cheek area and you may have some bruising. Applying ice and keeping your head elevated when reclining will help reduce the swelling. Chewing or brushing your teeth might be difficult for two weeks, but you may experience almost no discomfort. You may feel tightness or numbness around the treated area for a period of time.

Complications are rare. Antibiotics taken before and after the operation should prevent infection. Other complications can be avoided by following the directions given by your surgeon. Remember: Raising your blood pressure can cause a hematoma after *any* operation. Be smart and follow the general instructions for "Don'ts" in chapter 15. Don't smoke, or be around anyone who does.

A cheek implant can make a pretty woman prettier, and it may reduce the depth of nasolabial folds. The improvement is fabulous, and extremely lovely. So what's the catch?

Here's the trade-off.

Unless you have a narrow face, you may not see the results of your cheekbone implant for *six months*. Worse, if you have a round, full face to begin with, you may have fat "chipmunk cheeks" for a long time. The swelling associated with this operation lingers just enough so that you don't see that wonderfully sculpted look for months. You must be patient. Some girlfriends have insisted on removing the implants in three or four months because they hated the fullness in their cheeks. *Don't.* If you are going to do this procedure, plan on being a patient patient. You will see dramatic results; nearly 100 percent of girlfriends who did wait, loved the look they had . . . eventually. But you need to expect the wait!

Just Pucker . . . In Search of Lips

It's so depressing. Maybe you were born with thin lips. Maybe you had thin lips thrust upon you—because on top of everything else, aging leaves us with minimized lips, or virtually no lips at all. With plump lips now in fashion, even younger girlfriends want to increase their lip size. In fact, like Julia Roberts, some of us tried collagen shots. They are supposed to last two to three months. Hah! No girlfriend we know who has had collagen injections said it lasted that long. Susan said her collagen lasted just twenty-four hours. At $400 and up a treatment, that's a mighty expensive "temporary" solution.

The truth is that, because the lips move—in other words, they are dynamic—no injected solution to the problem is going to last.

There is help from implants. An implant of AlloDerm® seems to do a terrific job. Susan had this done, and the implant is totally invisible. Her lips swelled up a bit, not a lot, and were back to feeling normal in about a week. Her upper lip is definitely fuller, and she is happy with the results.

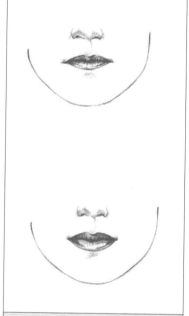

before/after lip supplementation

Chin Ups

The classical definition of a beautiful face is a face with perfect symmetry. The chin is essential in creating the balance of a lovely face. In fact, the chin must complement the nose, and often a chin implant will be recommended along with nose surgery. Sometimes, the chin implant alone will improve the nose's appearance.

Besides asymmetry, the problems of a weak chin, a double chin, or an overly strong chin can be eliminated with cosmetic surgery. And here's a bit of upsetting news: As you age, you may get a "witch's chin"!

"Witch's Chin"

"Witch's chin" is probably hereditary, since not every woman gets it. This growth and drooping of the end of the chin makes a girl-friend resemble the Wicked Witch in *The Wizard of Oz*. A number of procedures have been developed to correct this problem.

If you think you have "witch's chin," or might be developing it, look at yourself in profile and note whether the end of your chin droops down below the line of the jaw. If it does, don't get too upset. Not only can you get it fixed, some very famous *young* stars have it. Take a good look at Celine Dion! But don't despair, a "witch's chin" can be made to vanish, although it will take more than a wave of Glinda the Good Witch's wand; it takes a good plastic surgeon.

Chin Augmentation (Mentoplasty)

If you have a "weak" chin, or simply a chin that needs some augmentation to add better symmetry to the face, the development of chin implants has made this operation quick and easy. Another procedure, the one that doesn't use an implant, moves the chin bone forward. Still another may use a cartilage graft taken from your nose, if a rhinoplasty is being performed at the same time. Of all these, the chin implant is simplest.

The best candidate for chin augmentation is the individual with a receding chin and a normal dental bite. If you have a bite dysfunction, you will need jaw surgery along with the mentoplasty. However, some insurance companies will pay part or all of the costs of this surgery if the condition impairs normal jaw function.

The implant surgery can be done in a physician's office or a hospital, usually using local anesthetic and intravenous sedation. The incision is made either inside the mouth where there will be no visible scars, or under the chin. There are several sizes of implant, and it is placed in a pocket above the chin bone and beneath the muscles. A pressure bandage will be applied, and you will experience some swelling, and perhaps bruising.

If your own chin bone is used, it is moved forward from an incision inside the mouth. Special instruments cut through the chin bone, and the lower portion of the bone is then moved forward and wired to keep it in position. There is more pain associated with this operation than with an implant.

The bandages are removed in about a week. As with any surgical procedure, avoid any activities that can raise your blood pressure for at least two weeks, even though you will be up and around immediately after this procedure. (You can usually avoid hematomas if you take it easy.) Also, keeping your head elevated, and sleeping on your back on pillows, will help reduce swelling. Applying ice compresses also will reduce swelling. Chewing may be difficult for ten days to two weeks. Brushing your teeth may be difficult for a few days. Numbness around the treated area is normal, but sensation should return over time.

A chin implant offers nearly instant gratification and improvement in appearance. Also, if for any reason you don't like the implant, it is not difficult to remove. Beauty-contest winner Dina, who has a narrow face and chin, felt her smile was not as wide with the implant. She also said she could "feel" it. Although you should

---

MARILYN'S SECRET

As most people know, Marilyn Monroe did have a rhinoplasty. Few people realize, however, that in 1949 she had chin augmentation by plastic surgeon John Pangman, who performed a chin graft (Kron, *Lift*).

WHEN TO CALL YOUR DOCTOR

- If you experience significant pain.

- If you have sudden or unusual swelling.

- If you see signs of infection (pus, red streaks, heat around the wound).

wait six months before making any changes after *any* procedure, Dina decided rather quickly to have her implant removed. It was taken out with a local anesthetic, no pain, and virtually no recovery time. As she said, "It just popped out, and my chin went back to the way it had been. My mouth was a little sore, and that was it."

But girlfriends, remember to be a *patient* patient. Dina should have waited. Like cheek implants, chin implants cause swelling that lingers for months. You won't know if you love the look until *six months* have passed. *Wait!*

Double Chins (Redundant Chins)

Double chins respond beautifully to liposuction alone in younger women. Of course, liposuction combined with a face-lift results in a beautiful chin and jawline. (No more jowls!)

Strong Chin, or "Lantern Jaw"

Think Nurse Ratched in *One Flew Over the Cuckoo's Nest*. Think Jay Leno! His "lantern jaw" is part of his fame—but for a woman, a strong jaw may be part of her shame. A prominent, large jaw tends to make a woman look more masculine or tough, conveying the impression she is an unfeeling drill sergeant when she may be a sensitive artist. Surgery can correct a "strong" or oversized chin, but the specific procedure is dictated by the source of the problem and needs careful consultation with your surgeon. It can involve removing bone—or even teeth!

A LAST WORD ON ANCILLARY PROCEDURES WITH YOUR FACE-LIFT

To get total satisfaction and to get the beautiful results you want, face-lifts are nearly always combined with another procedure. You and your surgeon will discuss the options during your consultation. Ask questions, get clear answers, and don't be insulted if your doctor recommends a chin implant, remarks that your skin has been damaged by sun, or notes that your eyelids are drooping. *You are paying for expert advice, not flattery.*

If you do have severely wrinkled skin, you will need to combine your lift with some sort of resurfacing, usually by laser. Some of the early problems of combining laser and face-lifts have been eliminated, and *the combination is safe in the hands of an experienced surgeon.* Yes, the recovery time will be much longer, but a face-lift alone will not give you youthful-looking skin. Laser, or dermabrasion, at the same time as your lift is worth serious consideration if you have deep crow's-feet, lines around your lips, or those heavy "accordion" wrinkles (see section 4, "Getting the Wrinkles Out"). For the best rejuvenation money can buy, a face-lift and its associated procedures are a sure thing.

But wait! There is one major facial surgery we have left for last. Often performed on teenagers, it has to do with the facial feature that many women say they "hate": their nose. So read on to find out about . . . *nose jobs.*

9

NOSE JOBS!

Rhinoplasty has been around for a long time, described in the old-est known surgical record, on an ancient Egyptian papyrus (Adam-son, 93). If you hate your nose, it's nothing new to humankind. Look at the famous bust of Nefertiti. So, do you think she had a nose job?

Maybe your nose is too big, has a bump, is crooked, too flat, or droops—but whatever the problem, chances are, it has bothered you since adolescence. In fact, rhinoplasty is often performed in girls, after maturity, at fourteen or fifteen, and boys at fifteen to sixteen (Sheen, 153).

But no other plastic-surgery procedure carries as many emo-tional and psychological issues. Botched nose jobs have accounted for the murder of four plastic surgeons by disturbed male patients (Terino, 10). It is not uncommon for girlfriends to burst into tears when they first see their reconstructed nose. Cindy started sobbing when she saw her perfect "little" nose instead of the classic Roman nose that had dominated her delicate face for thirty years. "All I could think of was, 'I look like Michael Jackson!'"

One supermodel ran screaming from her plastic surgeon's office when she first saw the results. She called a few weeks later, raving about how much she loved it. Across the board there is an

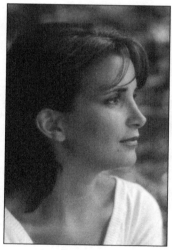

Cindy looks beautiful one year after her rhinoplasty.

acceptance curve, no matter how good a job a surgeon does. Your looks are profoundly and forever changed. When the bandages are first removed, your nose is pushed up, swollen, and far from what it will eventually look like. The most common reaction upon seeing a "fixed" nose for the first time after surgery is, "I've made the biggest mistake of my life."

Prepare yourself for the shock.

The Nose and Sex

Why do we react so strongly to changing our nose? Freud insisted our noses are tied to our sexuality, and you've probably heard that the size of a guy's nose is directly related to the size of his penis. (Hah, isn't that wishful thinking!) Also, our noses are often a badge of our ethnic background writ large on our face. Greek, Asian, African-American, Arab, or Hebrew—our nose proclaims our ancestry. Changing it can have deep psychological consequences. In short, there is no more worried, upset, neurotic, crazed, hopeful, tearful, and potentially out-of-control patient than one requesting a rhinoplasty. When it comes to pushing our buttons, the feature in the center of our face is directly connected to our very essence.

Are there botched nose jobs? You bet there are—lots. We'll try to give you some tips on how to avoid a bad rhinoplasty, but meanwhile, dear girlfriends, remember, a fine surgeon can usually fix a poor surgeon's mistakes.

PICKING A DOCTOR FOR YOUR NOSE JOB

Listen carefully:

- Not every plastic surgeon does a good nose.
- Not every good plastic surgeon can do the nose you want or need, and maybe no one can.

To discover how close your nose can come to an ideal nose, you need to find an experienced, artistically talented doctor. "Artistic"? Yes. One article says a doctor needs "to develop a sense of beauty, harmony, and proportion. . . . The beginning surgeon may find a course in the history of art a useful beginning for the appreciation of facial and body aesthetics" (Colton, 97).

A pleasing nose must fit your face, your height (a bigger person needs a bigger nose), and aspire to some objective standards of beauty about its length, its tip, and its shape. Girlfriends, we need to be totally blunt here: The "aesthetic norm" is a Caucasian nose. If you wish your nose to retain some ethnic identity, you need to make that clear with your doctor. Fixing your nose takes a great deal of measuring, thinking, and planning on the part of the doctor. And a great deal of talent.

To find the right doctor for your rhinoplasty, begin your evaluation with your consultation. It is said a good rhinoplastic surgeon needs a minimum of five years' experience, so you should ask how long the doctor has been doing this kind of surgery. You can find out how many rhinoplasties he or she performs a year. You can evaluate how thorough the consultation is, how well the doctor listens to your ideas, and what he or she says can be done or can't be done. Also, he or she should explain what the operation can accomplish, and how.

At this point, you need some education. *Read up before you go!* One thing you will discover is that there is a controversy raging between doctors who perform "open" surgeries and those who do "closed" surgeries. If the doctor suggests an "open" procedure, you will have visible scars, and perhaps an unsightly notch in the columella (the piece that separates your two nostrils, like a column holding up your nose's tip). A "closed" operation is done from inside the nose and doesn't leave a visible scar. One type of nose job that requires an open incision is making a wide nose narrower at the tip. Other types of repairs can usually be done with a closed

"I had a bump on my nose, and the bridge of my nose was always red. Although I used concealer to even out the tone to match the rest of my skin, makeup couldn't hide the bump! Every day I thought about my nose. I felt it didn't fit the rest of my face, which is small and fine-featured. For as long as I can remember, I avoided anyone seeing my profile. I'd carefully position myself so I directly faced anyone I was talking to. I never had a picture taken if I could avoid it. But the worst? Driving a car. Whenever I stopped at a red light, I put my hand up to cover my face because I knew people in nearby cars could see my profile. I never once got in the car without feeling miserable about it."

KAREN, PERSONAL TRAINER, RHINOPLASTY AT AGE THIRTY-FOUR

"My nose was too wide at the top. I felt like there was this huge 'thing' between my eyes. I liked everything about my face except that. It made me feel ugly. I was always aware of it, always thinking about it."

ANNE, OFFICE MANAGER,
RHINOPLASTY AT AGE
FORTY-ONE

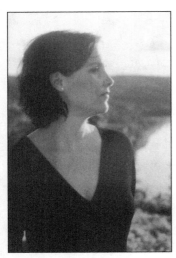

Anne looks and feels wonderful as a result of her surgery.

procedure. If the surgeon says you need an open approach, please get a second opinion just to be sure.

Most important, if you can't see any noses in person (ask if anyone on the nursing or office staff has had a rhinoplasty by the doctor), ask to see lots of photos of noses the doctor has fixed. See if you like his or her work. Notice whether all the noses look similar (some doctors only do "one nose"), or if the noses vary with the individuals. Look for a patient with a nose like yours and see what kind of results that person had. Even if you have to pay for more than one consultation, don't settle for anything less than a doctor with whom you feel total confidence.

Even after you make a wise choice, even with the very best doctor, some girlfriends still need a second surgery for revisions because no one can predict exactly how a nose will heal.

The procedure.

Rhinoplasty can be performed in a physician's office, an outpatient surgical facility, or a hospital. It may be done under general anesthesia, but it is also performed under local anesthetic and intravenous sedation. An operation that includes a septoplasty may be covered by insurance. It is done in the hospital.

To remove a hump in your nose, a special file or chisel is used. A narrower nasal bridge is then formed by bringing together the bones on either side of the face. In patients in whom the size of the nasal tip is too large, cartilage is removed through an incision inside the nose. The angle between the nose and the upper lip can be improved by elevating and trimming the septum, which is the dividing wall between the two chambers of the nose. A "deviated septum" is one that has moved to the side and is hampering your breathing.

If it is necessary to narrow the base of the nose, skin has to be removed from both sides of the nostrils. In order to improve the contour of the noses of some patients, it is sometimes necessary to add tissue. Where does this tissue come from? Probably your ear!

No matter what your problem, there is a technique developed to fix it. But, remember girlfriends, rhinoplasties are considered the "queens" of plastic-surgery operations because they test a surgeon's skill. A rhinoplasty needs more than a surgeon's competence; as we said before, a rhinoplasty requires an artist's hand.

Recovery from a Rhinoplasty

First of all, a lightweight splint is applied to the top of the nose to keep the shape in place during healing. It's held on with adhesive tape—very noticeable, unmistakable white tape. Not only is your nose now a beacon in the night, the splint can have an unexpected impact. As long as Karen had the splint on, she had episodes of fainting. While the doctor removed it, she went dead white and nearly passed out. As soon as the splint came off, she was fine. We don't know why this happens, but be aware that for some reason the pressure of the splint can cause this—and you need to exercise caution to prevent a fall. The splint comes off in about a week.

Packing is inserted in the nose to protect the septum after surgery. It does not feel good at all, and getting it removed after three to five days is a blessed relief. Also, you will have a "mustache" bandage under your nose to keep drainage from running down your face. You will have to change it until it, too, is removed, when you stop dripping.

The stitches inside the nose will dissolve. Any outside the nose will need to be removed one week after surgery.

Girlfriend-to-Girlfriend Tips

Your surgeon will give you post-operative instructions; be sure to read them and follow them carefully. *Don't do anything on your own or because that's what a friend did.*

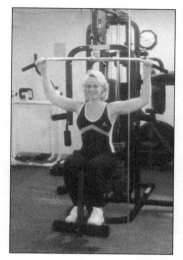

Karen's rhinoplasty has given her a reason to smile.

Special don'ts for a rhinoplasty, straight from girlfriends who've been there.

• Do not sneeze. If you can't help but sneeze, let the air out through your mouth, not your nose. If you feel the urge to sneeze, press your finger on your upper lip and this may inhibit the impulse. The problem is, girlfriends, you may not feel the sneeze coming on. Don't be polite—let it out through your mouth!

• Do not blow your nose. You will want to . . . oh, will you want to! You absolutely *should not* do it. You will feel congested, uncomfortable, even downright miserable. Distract yourself. Try to think about something else. You cannot blow your nose until the doctor says you can—after about *six weeks*. Gently use a Q-Tip with saline spray to remove excessive dry mucus from inside the nose. Keeping hydrated (drink lots of water!) will help relieve some of the feelings of congestion.

• Do not pick your nose. If you are a secret nose-picker, this message is meant for you. You will want to because of those darn crusts. *Don't.* Start knitting or crocheting if you can't stop picking.

• Do not touch your nose. Keep your fingers away from the area as much as possible.

• Do not set your eyeglasses on your nose. Tape them to your forehead for two weeks after the surgery. However, you *can* wear contact lenses as soon as your eyes feel normal (no swelling).

• Do not lift children! Cindy notes that if you have children under two, *do not get a rhinoplasty.* You should not hold any children who will be grabbing at your nose or may hit your nose with their head or a toy.

• Do not get into a major fight with a significant other. Fortunately, for the first forty-eight hours you aren't capable of arguing. But, if you have a rocky home situation, go else-where. *Figure this out before the operation.* Face reality. *Don't* put yourself in a situation where you'll get upset. Don't let your-self start crying. You know how your nose runs when you cry? You don't need that extra drainage after a rhinoplasty.

Seeing the light of day after surgery.

Expect to be noticed if you venture from the house while you still have the splint and big white bandages on. (Consider others, and don't go out while your nose is draining and you still have the mustache bandage on.) If you have opted to tell a cover story instead of saying you had rhinoplasty, you can say you had a deviated septum, or a broken nose from being hit with a tennis racket, oar, softball, or golf club. (Pick your favorite sport. Bowl-ing probably won't work though.) You can say you had an acci-dent. Remember the air-bag lie (see chapter 7, on face-lifts if you didn't see it). But heed the first rule of lying: You can say anything, no matter how outrageous, and people will believe you if you say it with sincerity and conviction. But keep your explanation short and simple. Long, elaborate stories always sound defensive and phony.

Also, be sure you heed the following advice.

- Wear a sunblock with SPF 15 or above around your eyes and nose until all the bruising is gone—*and on all incisions for a minimum of four to six months after surgery.* The sun interferes with healing and may cause excessive redness and itching. It can also cause hyperpigmentation (darker skin), which will take longer to fade.

- Makeup can be applied everywhere but your nose. After the splint is removed, use hypoallergenic paramedical makeup products (see list on page 197). They are usually well-tolerated and are effective as cover-ups. If you had any incisions,

"As long as my husband was alive, I couldn't do anything about the bump on my nose. 'Angie,' he'd say, 'I married that nose, and you're not going to change it.' I had broken my nose when I was six years old. It was never right after that, and I suf-fered horrible headaches all my life. Finally, when I decided to have a face-lift, I asked the sur-geon about my nose. He felt that there was definitely damage, and he could help me. After the surgery was over, he said the amount of scar tissue he removed was enormous. I was very pleased with the appearance of my 'new' nose, and best of all, it's been ten years—and I have never had another of those headaches."

ANGIE, HOMEMAKER,
RHINOPLASTY AT AGE
SIXTY-THREE

remember that makeup becomes contaminated. *Don't use it on an unhealed incision.* And expect the problems of putting on makeup over flaky skin, because you will have peeling after the swelling goes down.

What to Expect Medically After Rhinoplasty

- Vomiting or coughing up old blood immediately after surgery. This does not happen to everyone, but sometimes you will have blood in your stomach from the surgery. It is not something to be concerned about unless you vomit repeatedly—then call the doctor.

- A small amount of bloody drainage for three to five days after the surgery. Change the mustache dressing under your nose as necessary.

- Crust or dried blood inside the nose after the packing is removed. See the directions for cleaning it in text above.

- Swelling inside the nose. If this persists, you will probably be prescribed a nasal steroid spray called Vancenase.

- Swelling on the tip of the nose. If this occurs, tell your doctor. This may require a steroid shot.

- Bruising (black eyes) and swelling. The discoloration will become more noticeable on the second or third day after surgery. Diligent application of ice packs, oral vitamin C, arnica montana, and vitamin K cream will speed healing. Normally, bruising is completely resolved by three weeks.

- Discomfort, and mild to moderate pain. This should be readily alleviated by Darvocet or Tylenol No.3.

- Congestion, or difficulty breathing through your nose after the packing is removed. This should go away on its own as the swelling subsides, but if the feeling persists, talk to your doctor.

Some girlfriends felt they were more prone to sinus infections after having a rhinoplasty.

It takes six to twelve months for nasal swelling to completely disappear. Expect to see gradual improvement for three to six months. As healing continues, the final result will emerge. The results of this surgery can be dramatic or spectacular, but *you must be patient during the healing phase. Do not consider corrections or changes until after six months have passed.*

COMPLICATIONS

Serious, life-threatening complications are rare after a rhinoplasty. More common medical complications include the following.

- Headache or fainting. The pressure of the splint causes this in some people.

- Infection. A possibility, but unlikely because you are probably receiving antibiotics for five days after surgery.

- Hematoma or seroma. There is a remote possibility that some blood or serum may collect under the skin. If it occurs, it can usually be evacuated in the doctor's office. Occasionally, a patient may require a return to the operating room for treatment.

- Altered sense of smell, temporarily or permanently. You might not be able to smell odors or taste food—or taste it as well—after surgery. This may be a result of congestion, and it's usually temporary. However, there is a remote possibility that the loss could be permanent.

- Red-nose syndrome. A worsening of telangiectasis—redness—on the bridge of the nose.

- Injury to the tear ducts. Tear ducts may not work properly, or your eyes will tear too much. If the condition doesn't

WHEN TO CALL YOUR DOCTOR

- If there is excessive bleeding or if the mustache dressing must be changed more than two to three times per hour for two to three hours in a row.

- If there is blood running down the back of your throat, making it difficult to breathe or swallow.

- If you experience significant or constant pain.

- If swelling increases, if an area of the face becomes swollen and hard, or if you develop a fever.

resolve on its own, you will probably be referred to an eye specialist.

- Runny nose. Some girlfriends complained that their noses seemed to start running spontaneously and without warning after their rhinoplasties. That well may be, but we hate to tell you, girlfriends, it also happens as you age.

- Mucous cyst. Although rare, this can happen years after the surgery, and it appears as a swelling mass on the nose (Kotzur, 520).

- Nasal collapse. This also can happen over time, and a depression on the ridge of the nose or a "ski nose" results.

- Notched columella. This unsightly notch, which will mar your profile, is the result of open surgery.

- Fracture. Athletes, especially, must be very careful to avoid injury to their nose after a rhinoplasty. During the first six weeks after surgery it is very fragile. Even later, a nose, after rhinoplasty, is more easily fractured (Guyuron, 313).

But, more common than medical complications are less-than-great results such as the following.

- Nose too small.

- Nose not small enough.

- Tip not refined enough.

- Notch in the tip.

- Permanent asymmetry in the nostril or the bridge of nose appears off to one side. Try to remember while you are staring at yourself that no nose is perfectly symmetrical. Your nostrils will be a bit uneven; you may think your nose is crooked. Check your "before" pictures and try to stay objective. If it's a bad job (it happens), seek a second opinion. Some patients see several doctors and have several operations before they are satisfied. However, continued dissatisfaction with a rhinoplasty that looks good to everyone else may be a symptom of an emotional and psychological problem.

Another look at your chin.

A rhinoplasty is often combined with a chin implant. They go together like yin and yang. Your chin and nose should be in balance. If your surgeon suggests an implant, you should listen carefully, weigh the pros and cons, and make your own decision. Without the implant, you may not see the results you want.

A FINAL WORD ON THE SCHNOZZ

Few people ever regret getting a nose job. The only exceptions occur if they had the operation in their teens and now—their values having changed—wish they had kept a more "ethnic" nose. But that is hindsight. At the time, their nose made them miserable.

One more depressing fact about aging: Your nose, like your chin, can grow as the years roll by. In some people, it becomes a serious problem, a "witch's nose" to match the "witch's chin." Rhinoplasty makes the problem vanish . . . with a sincere wish, "two clicks of the ruby slippers," and a wonderful plastic surgeon.

If you desire a nose job—if it is a longing deep and dear, girlfriend—*do it.*

GETTING THE WRINKLES OUT

LASER:
A BURNING SENSATION

We all hate lines and wrinkles! We use lotions, go to salons for facials, or look hideous in mud masks—all in pursuit of youthful skin. But aside from Retin-A, alpha-hydroxy or glycolic peels and products, those over-the-counter beauty products will moisturize with the same efficiency as Vaseline or Crisco, but they won't do a doggone thing to eliminate wrinkles or change our skin. Beauty products sell us hope, take our money, and leave us disappointed.

Of course, you do have it within your power to maintain your skin without pain, risk, and at very little cost. In fact, you may save money and improve your health. Here are the facts, in a nutshell.

- First, if you smoke, stop. It ruins your skin.

- Second, stay out of the sun *and tanning booths*. As much as 96 percent of the visible signs of aging are a result of cumulative sun damage. "What damage?" Honey, hold on, here's the list of uglies: fine lines, wrinkles (including skin that looks like an alligator's), textural changes, brown spots, elastosis (loss of elasticity), coarse dryness, blood-vessel damage, skin growths, breakdown of collagen, and yellow or gray skin tinges, due to a loss of blood vessels that provide circulation to the surface of the skin. As much as 80 percent of the damage may come from sun exposure you had before the age of ten!

Protecting your skin isn't hard to do: Use opaque clothing, sunblock, and/or sunscreen anytime you're outdoors. Sun damage is not a joke, and you can't "get away with it." If you are fair-skinned and of Northern European descent, you may see lines around your mouth and eyes in your twenties, serious wrinkles in your thirties, and be at high risk for skin cancer at any time.

- Third, drink in moderation, and don't do drugs at all. Too much alcohol will cause what is called telangiectasia, or reddish noses and cheeks filled with broken veins.

- Fourth, eat nutritious food and take a good supplement formulated for skin that includes beta-carotene (or better yet, a combination of carotenes), vitamin C, horsetail grass, and gotu kola. Good nutrition and nutritional supplements will help your skin stay healthy, more youthful, and heal faster.

But how do you get rid of the damaged skin and wrinkles you already have? You have some options and, in almost every case, a hard choice to make.

LASER: EMBRACE THE LIGHT— BUT DO IT CAREFULLY

No more acne scars, accordion-like wrinkles, lines around the eyes and mouth, wine-stain birthmarks, scars, sagging skin . . . Can laser really perform these skin miracles? From what we've experienced, studied, seen, read, and heard from other women, the answer is a cautious, "Yes, but . . ." What is the "but" all about? The most common complaint is the extraordinarily long healing process. Second is the risk of a complication like hyperpigmentation (dark patches), hypopigmentation (light or white areas), and scarring.

With laser resurfacing, as in *most* plastic surgeries done for cosmetic reasons, the results of a procedure come with a trade-off. You get what you want, but you get something you don't want at the same time. When it comes to laser treatments, the trade-off can be a tough call. Nevertheless, in 1998, 123,666 people underwent laser skin-resurfacing to get that youthful look (American Society for Aesthetic Plastic Surgery).

When things go well with laser, as they do most of the time, truly youthful skin is the wonderful bonus. Besides removing wrinkles and imperfections, laser tightens the underlying collagen and improves the elasticity of the skin. But are you willing to stay indoors looking like Lon Chaney as "The Mummy" for up to two weeks? Are you ready to cover redness with makeup for several months, and maybe up to a year? And worse—if you *do* have a complication, the truth is, you will be scared silly. In fact, since this is your face, and even a pimple sends most of us into a tailspin, a laser complication will bring you the mother of all anxiety attacks. You will feel as if you will never look like yourself again; you may even become distraught. (Rest assured, in nearly every case, your doctor and time will put things right.) Plus, any complication means you must endure an even a longer recovery period. That, girlfriends, is the real deal you need to consider *before* you decide to do a fast, not a slow burn.

What laser is.

The word *laser* comes from an acronym for "light amplification by the stimulated emission of radiation." The laser vaporizes skin cells one layer at a time; in theory, without bleeding (in reality, you might bleed a lot). Vaporizing layers of skin just four or five cells in thickness, the laser preserves the underlying skin tissue.

Unlike dermabrasion and chemical peels, where penetration can be unpredictable, laser's technology and the visual clues it gives as it vaporizes your skin, lets your doctor control exactly how deeply the laser penetrates.

As with all procedures, you will have an initial consultation with your doctor. Come prepared, with specific questions to ask. Discuss anything that concerns you. Be sure to get clear answers as to what outcome you can expect. For example, if you wish to remove acne scars, get a realistic idea of how much of the scarring laser can remove.

Controversy still rages about what is the best way to prepare for laser resurfacing. Most doctors develop their own instructions for you to follow. Current wisdom is to do as little as possible—but that approach may change as testing continues and new products are developed.

The procedure is usually performed in the physician's office. A local anesthetic and intravenous sedation provide the best assurance that you will feel no pain. Topical anesthetics alone probably won't be enough. The specific areas that you want treated, such as the crow's-feet around your eyes or scarring on your cheeks, will usually receive more than one pass of the laser. Please be realistic about the outcome. You will likely see a dramatic improvement—but not perfect skin. If you are having a full-face laser resurfacing,

QUESTIONABLE DOCTOR ALERT

Girlfriends, we recently saw an ad for laser resurfacing in our local "freebie" paper—the one that gives the counterculture horoscope and reviews the latest music releases. No credentials for the "doctor" were given. The ad was big, bold, and tempting. And dangerously seductive. While any MD is legally allowed to purchase a machine and perform laser resurfacing, not just any MD should do it. Review chapter 13, "Finding a Doctor." We recommend that your laser resurfacing should be done only by a board-certified plastic surgeon or a board-certified dermatologist, both of whom are experts in skin-related treatments.

the areas you want treated (around your eyes, mouth, or over your cheeks), will get several passes of the laser. The smoother areas of your face might receive just one pass of the laser, or a "feather-touch." "Feather-touch" is a lighter "dose" of laser, with the machine set at a lower power.

Afterward your face may be covered in a special kind of flesh-tone, adhesive bandages (the most common one used is Flexzan) for seven to ten days. There is usually no pain while the bandages are on. Only when areas are exposed to the air will you feel pain, or as if your face is "burning." Girlfriend Denise described the feeling when her bandages were removed and air hit her face as a "twang" for a few seconds that quickly went away. Susan described it as a "blast of pain." Pauline called it "excruciating."

Some doctors prefer open treatment (no bandages). When there is nothing covering your treated skin, you must keep the area constantly moist with compresses and moisturizers. Drying, crusting, and scabbing should be avoided, and you should be told how to clean and care for your skin.

If you don't get clear written instructions, ask! If you have questions after you go home, call the doctor's office and ask. *Don't try anything on your own. If you develop intense pain, call your doctor.* Don't be hesitant about having your concerns addressed. It's your face!

What you see (at first) is not what you get.

Everyone stares at Pauline's skin. It looks as smooth as fresh cream. She's one of those women who has a complexion to die for, and it's a beautiful part of her entire look, from her gamine face and red hair, to her wonderfully tailored clothes. Hardworking, independent, and assertive, she looks as if she's in her early thirties; she just passed the big four-oh. Her gorgeous skin is less than a year old . . . because Pauline got the look with laser. When Pauline had her bandages removed a week after surgery, this is what she described:

When I was handed the mirror, I was not prepared for what I saw. My heart went straight to my toes. (Nor was I prepared for the pain over the next twenty-four hours!) My face was still very swollen and bright red. Even though I had seen pictures of other patients to prepare me, I was shocked at how I looked. There were some dark red open areas, and my chin area looked different than the rest of my face. I later learned a "feather-touch" was used on parts of my face, and more intense laser on others. I was told to be concerned only if I developed "lesions."

That night it felt as if my face were oozing. When I woke up, I had a whitish yellow oozing patch on my right cheek. Was this a lesion? I called the doctor's office and was told this was normal. But I also had "fish-scale"–looking marks on my forehead that didn't come off. I had an area that was raised and looked like a "floating island." I felt very upset and anxious because I didn't know what was normal and what wasn't. I also didn't know it was going to look as bad as it did. All of the oozing and deep redness disappeared in a week, and I was amazed at the healing powers of my body. I'm also pleased with my results.

If you do not have dressings on your skin, but are healing with the open-wound technique, then your skin will produce "exudate" (a yellowish substance) that can last seven days after a light laser treatment, and ten to fourteen days after deeper treatments. Like Pauline, you may wonder if it is pus and if the discharge is normal. If you are concerned, call your doctor (panel discussion, page 122). The oozing is removed by gentle cleansing and then keeping the skin moist. You need to wash with the gentle cleanser that your doctor recommends and gently pat dry. *Do not rub the skin.* Wetting and rinsing can be accomplished with a splashing motion. Cool water will feel refreshing and soothing.

How red are you? "Coca-Cola Classic®" can red. This bright redness can last for six to eight weeks. The color will steadily fade to pink, but it may be a year before the pink disappears entirely. You may have a sensation of excessive tightness from the third through eighth weeks after surgery (Achauer, 32–34). *Any intense pain, however, is not normal. It may be a sign of infection. Let your doctor know right away!*

Things you need to know before you go.

- Because laser resurfacing is a relatively new technique, there is still controversy over the best ways to prepare the patient in the weeks before the procedure, and even what to do afterwards. Generally, it is agreed that you should be given an anti-herpes medication before the surgery because the procedure can bring on an outbreak of herpes, even in some patients who have not experienced it before. You might want to research this in the library or on-line, because new studies are being done all the time on the most effective treatments. Then you can discuss what you read with your doctor. However, no matter what you find on your own, follow your practitioner's instructions to the letter. *Don't take or apply anything on your own!*

- Laser works best on wrinkles caused by sun damage rather than wrinkles caused by movement (called "dynamic" wrinkles), because the latter will eventually come back. However, some

---

A TIP TO REMEMBER

Here is an invaluable tip about any cream, ointment, makeup—about *anything* you put on your face. Sometimes you may experience a mild stinging for a few seconds. But listen carefully: Any stinging that lasts for more than a few seconds is not normal. Any pain is not normal. Do *not* tough it out. Do *not* be a trouper. Get whatever you put on your face off by rinsing with cool water. Continue flushing your face with water until the stinging stops. If the stinging or pain persists, call your doctor or seek help.

dynamic wrinkles can now be prevented with Botox (see pages 215–17), and laser works effectively to diminish the remaining lines, such as the frown lines between your eyes. Laser excels at eliminating crow's-feet and getting rid of wrinkles under the eyes. Pitted acne scars and irregular skin texture will disappear dramatically—from 25 to 50 percent—but not entirely. "Ice pick" scars or deeper pits, however, need to be surgically removed (Weinstein et al, pages 216–25).

Interestingly, if you are in your seventies or eighties, you may have the most spectacular results of all, with noticeable tightening of the skin, a youthful appearance, and no more wrinkles. However, laser will not remove jowls, bags under the eyes, or other problems of excess skin such as wattles or crepe neck.

- Laser will likely cause scarring if done on the neck, back, or hands. It's been tried, and it's too risky.

- Moles and other possible cancerous growths can be removed by laser—but not biopsied (because they are vaporized). For that reason, laser is not a good choice for any bump, mole, or mark that could be cancerous or pre-cancerous (*Self*, page 131).

DON'T PICK—DON'T SCRATCH

If you do have scabs or crusts, it is very important that you don't pick at them. "Secret" face-pickers—you know who you are, you girlfriends who pick and squeeze in front of the bathroom mirror, then try to cover up the evidence with cold compresses and makeup—take note! You will cause scarring.

Also, if you experience itching, *don't scratch*. Ask your doctor what you can do to relieve it. You may be reacting to a topical medication. Usually hydrocortisone cream will end the problem (Weinstein et al, 221). Don't put anything on your face without your doctor's approval.

Also, try to sleep on your back. Even rubbing your face against the pillow can cause redness from broken capillaries under the skin (telangiectasia) (Weinstein, 223–24). If this happens, girlfriends, remember, this is temporary!

- Your skin type and many other factors will greatly influence your reaction and results. Dark skin is difficult to correct by any means, and African-American women might look into microdermabrasion (see pages 207–8) if laser looks too risky. Skin that has darkened from repeated sun exposure will heal at a lighter tone than untreated skin.

- You might consider a full-face laser even if you need work only on a small area. The demarcation line where the laser stops and untreated skin begins is hard to cover with makeup. Since it is far easier to camouflage redness on the entire face, it might be better to get a feather-touch on the full face. In fact, people will think you simply have a sunburn, if they notice at all. However, the major exception to this suggestion is laser done on crow's-feet and under the eyes. This area is easy to camouflage. Want "eyes à la carte"? Go for it.

- If you are prone to acne, you might get an outbreak or lots of little whiteheads (milia) after the procedure (Weinstein, 221). Discuss this with your doctor so that you are given a non-greasy moisturizer to use following surgery. If you do get an outbreak, tell your doctor. It can be treated easily with topical creams, or even oral medication. But if you don't treat it, you might end up with new scars—and wouldn't that be ironic, and terribly disappointing.

- Fungal, or *Candida*, infections can occur with the use of some ointments—or if you live in a warm, hot, humid climate such as south Florida (panel discussion, page 121).

- Hyperpigmentation, or darker skin, is normal after laser resurfacing (Weinstein, 220). Most of the time it is temporary, but it can last many months and make you very unhappy. Your practitioner can give you bleaching creams to use at home. Don't panic and think you will always have the problem. Talk over your concerns with your doctor or the nurses. *Follow instructions*

ACCUTANE WARNING

If you have been taking Accutane for up to eighteen months prior to surgery, tell your doctor. It can retard healing and lead to scarring. This is also true if you are considering dermabrasion (Apfelberg, 1822–23).

for using creams to the letter, and don't put anything on your skin without your doctor's approval.

- Hypopigmentation (lighter skin) may not be noticeable until six months or more after surgery. It is usually permanent (Weinstein, 221).

Being seen in public after laser resurfacing.

Before you venture into the world, you need camouflage! You must ask your doctor when you can begin using makeup, but generally it will be between ten to fourteen days *after* the procedure. Before that, to be honest, expect to stay home and be told to keep your skin moist with Crisco (we kid you not!), petrolatum (Vaseline), Aguafor, Eutra, squaline, Hydrotone, or Bag Balm. *Do not put anything on your face that the doctor has not approved.* We can't stress that strongly enough. Even if you are sure it's okay, even if your best friend used it, *don't*. The consequences can be dreadful!

When you get the okay, you can use special camouflage makeup to cover up the redness. Susan's salon, Age of Innocence™, has

---

SUN EXPOSURE ALERT

Laser resurfacing removes the protective barrier provided by the upper layers of the skin. You can go outdoors two weeks after your procedure, but you *must avoid direct sun exposure* for four to six months until your normal skin color returns. Going outdoors means just walking to your car, too! You must be protected against any exposure. Use sunblock with SPF 15 to 30, and a hat and/or large sunglasses (Seckel). A brand of sunblock you might try is Glyderm Super Sunblock SPF 25. Another is Jan Marini Daily Face Protectant SPF 30 Waterproof Antioxidant. Both are very emollient and will aid in moisturizing the affected areas.

If you were a sun-worshipper and loved the look of a tan, your skin no longer has the pigmentation to tan. Be grateful you are not even tempted to risk skin cancer anymore. If you want the look, use a sunless self-tanner. In recent years they are much improved (no more orange!) and easy once you get the knack of applying them. We've used the Jan Marini product and were pleased, but there are dozens of very good ones on the market.

its own brand of paramedical makeup. The term "paramedical" describes the type of makeup you need, and you can use the term when you ask for it. You also want a brand that is not heavy like stage makeup, but lighter. Susan's paramedical line, and many others, have foundations with a green, purple, or yellow base, which you apply to "cancel out" the red. Different colors work on different shades of "wounded" complexions ranging from red to purple. This colored foundation will come in a compact, stick, tube, or lotion. Over the green, purple, or yellow base, you will put the skin-toned makeup, which is somewhat heavier than you would use normally. With Age of Innocence paramedical makeup, you finish with a powder, which fixes the makeup in place (it chemically interacts with the creamy makeup). The technique for applying a paramedical makeup is different from everyday makeup, so you need to get help from a professional to get the best results. When you buy the product, ask if someone is available to help you.

Susan's Story

To see Susan without makeup today, you would see a fair-skinned, beautiful green-eyed blonde with a fresh complexion. You would have to look very closely to see the tiny scars and blotchy spots on the sides of her face and on her forehead. In fact, you might not see them at all. Instead, you'd notice that her skin is elastic and toned, without a wrinkle in sight. Her fair, lovely skin is what you might expect to see on a young woman in her twenties. But there was a time after her laser procedure when Susan wondered if she'd ever look normal again. Here's her story. . . .

> When laser resurfacing was just beginning to be popular in the early 1990s, I was going to have the procedure, as a guinea pig. I thought the results looked astonishing. But I

knew I wasn't an ideal candidate. I have extremely fair skin, and I tend to get blotchy if I go out in the sun. I also had gotten the classic "mask of pregnancy" when I had both of my children. Then I went to a conference on laser complications and saw people so horribly scarred they looked like burn victims. I thought, *Oh no, I'm not going to risk that.*

But as time passed, the medical profession learned a great deal about using laser safely. After our office had handled between eighty and one hundred clients with great results and no major complications, I changed my mind again. I wanted to smooth out my skin and, especially, get rid of some crow's-feet around my eyes. Because of my skin type, however, I was going to get an extremely light resurfacing around my eyes and on my forehead, and a "feather-touch" over my full face.

Everything went great. And when the bandages were on, I had no pain at all. However, the minute the Flexzan was removed and air hit my face, I experienced a shockingly intense pain.

For the first three weeks, I healed beautifully. My skin re-epithelialized [grew back] quickly. The bright redness was fading, and I thought I was in the clear. Then three weeks after the procedure, my skin started getting darker. It was the complication I had worried about—hyperpigmentation. So I went to the medical chest and took out the bleaching agent that is recommended in all the literature, hydroquinone. I stood in front of the mirror and rubbed it on my face. Immediately I felt burning. I thought it would stop. It didn't. Even with my medical background, I ignored what my body was telling me. I was going to be stoic. I was going to tough it out because the hydroquinone was "good for me." The burning feeling didn't stop. I didn't know it, but I was getting a chemical burn on top of the laser burn.

I still remember getting into the car to drive home that day. It was summer, and the sun was coming through the windshield. When the sun hit my face, I felt as if my face were on fire. I put the pedal to the floor and raced to get home and put ice cubes on my face.

Once I made it home after a white-knuckled ride, I kept the ice cubes on my face continuously. As soon as they melted, I kept getting more from the freezer. As long as the coldness was on my skin, I couldn't feel the burning. But when you have laser, you feel a tight feeling that is indescribable. You have to moisturize your skin constantly. So finally, I had to put Vaseline on because my skin felt so taut. But I knew something was wrong. *And then, later, I put the hydroquinone on again.* Why? I thought I was doing the

PARAMEDICAL MAKEUP PRODUCTS FOR POST-LASER RESURFACING

- Physician's Formula. Find it by calling 1-800-227-0333; it is available in most drugstores.

- Estee Lauder. Available in department stores.

- Mary Kay Cosmetics. Full-coverage concealer.

- Shiseido. Stick foundation and powder compact.

- Chanel's Teint Extrême Lumière.

- Adrian Arpel. Blue concealer tube.

- Ultima II (Revlon) Aqua Tint.

- Huma Tech. Laser kit.

- Age of Innocence. Call with questions, or order it at (570) 674-5555, or on-line at www.skincaresalon.com.

(O'Donoghue, 717–18)

right thing. I didn't talk to my husband about it, and I should have. It was incredibly foolish.

Within two days, my skin began tightening so much that my lower eyelids were pulled down until the pink showed. Not only did my eyelids droop horribly, my mouth was pulled down and distorted. Then, my whole face began to contort. Soon I looked like a burn victim. I immediately began to see specialists. They all said they thought my face would heal—in time. They all explained that the skin heals from the inside out. The last dermatologist I saw assured me my face wouldn't peel; that healing would be gradual.

That night my skin started coming off in sheets, and my face immediately went back to normal. The pulling was gone. I can't explain my relief. My face looked like raw hamburger, literally. The laser resurfacing procedure was perfect. But my skin had had a reaction to the bleaching agent. Later, I found I was allergic.

In fact, I got through the experience better than my family, who were all very upset. Whenever I confront something really difficult, like this, the way I cope is to think that things could be worse. I think that at least my children are okay and nothing else is more important. All during this experience, I never got angry. I never blamed anyone. I believed my face would heal in time. But after the "hamburger" lesions healed, my skin looked like an orange peel! I used a lot of cover stick that entire summer. After three years, I still saw improvement every month.

Would I do it again? I love the results now, and I'm not sorry I did it. But if I had it to do over, no, I wouldn't do it. Even if I didn't have complications, the recovery period is just too long for me.

Now it's your call, we think . . .

Many people have great results from laser resurfacing. Several of the women we talked to love the way their skin looks. Certainly, if you feel bad about yourself every time you look in the mirror, and your doctor says laser will help you, you have a compelling reason to do it. If you have very wrinkled, alligator-like facial skin, laser is one of the best ways to treat the problem. Only *you* know the intensity of your feelings about the cosmetic problem that is bothering you. If you have a problem or imperfection that is hurting you deeply, then the risk and discomfort from laser resurfacing are justified. In fact, when laser is good, it is very, very good; but, like the little girl with the curl in the middle of her forehead, when laser is bad, it's horrid.

BAG BALM—IT'S UDDERLY WONDERFUL

In the familiar green can (well, it's familiar if you grew up on a dairy farm), Bag Balm is a safe, inexpensive moisturizer to apply after laser surgery—even though it was developed for a cow's udder. The directions say, "After each milking, apply thoroughly and allow coating to remain on the surface." Since 1899, Bag Balm has been the farmer's friend. Of course, people soon found out it worked on their skin too, and the company started putting out a "purse size" one-ounce version of the ten-ounce can at a premium price. But get the bigger ten-ounce size can at a large pet-supply store; it costs about $7. It's a mix of lanolin and petroleum jelly (so if you have a wool allergy, don't use it), very soft in consistency, and very moisturizing. Its big drawback? It smells like wet, unbleached wool. But you don't want perfumes or dyes on your face right now, so Bag Balm is a *moo*-velous choice.

A KINDER, GENTLER LASER . . . TO GET RID OF UNWANTED HAIR

Do you have a mustache, and you don't want to look like Groucho? Girlfriend Flossy—a feisty, blue-eyed athlete—did. Now, she has an upper lip as smooth as a baby's bottom. She swears that "photo-epilation" (this hair-removal laser is also called EpiLaser, SoftLight, or EpiLight) is the greatest invention since pantyhose.

I was told the EpiLight would take three treatments to eliminate my mustache. By the last treatment all I had left was a fine down above my upper lip. It didn't hurt at all. The process was as quick and fast as the popping of an old-fashioned flashbulb. First, the nurse rubbed a gel on the hair to be removed. She put the machine in place, and *presto!* I wasn't even uncomfortable, but I did smell singed hair!

This system leaves electrolysis in the dark ages, along with the waxing I endured for years. I hated waxing so much I'd rather have a root canal. Just anticipating that pain had me tense. After putting the hot wax on, they'd tell me, "Oh, it's only a little pinch." And waxing left me red and sore. Now that's a fading memory. I figure, with all the money I spent on waxing over the years, I'll even end up ahead financially.

However, the process does not guarantee complete hair removal, only 50 to 60 percent. Nor does it promise that the hair won't grow back after a number of months. But the initial feedback from women who have had it done has been raves. Some of them had tried electrolysis, which was painful, painstaking, and 50 percent of the hair did grow back. Plus, electrolysis can leave holes, significant redness, and cause infection. Photo-epilation doesn't have those risks.

What risks does photo-epilation pose?

They are minimal, but aftereffects can include reddening, mild burning, temporary bruising, and temporary discoloration of the skin.

One problem with the process: It works best on darker hair against lighter skin. White hairs are nearly impossible to remove since the laser is attracted to the melanin (the pigment) in the hair.

Coarse hairs, like those chin hairs we hate, are tougher to eliminate, and take more sessions. Blonde hair is stubborn, too, though better techniques are overcoming this drawback.

Women (and men) who get the best results fastest are people who tend to sunburn rather than tan (less melanin in the skin). Those who tan more easily tend to have more variation in their results. Despite those cautions, for anyone with excessive hair on any part of their body, this procedure, which covers large areas fast, and virtually painlessly, is a blessing.

So what's the price tag?

Photo-epilation is not cheap but it is affordable. You may have to compare prices, because they can vary widely. Of course, be sure you are going to a reputable office (one offered in conjunction with the office of a board-certified plastic surgeon or dermatologist is certainly safest). Some sample prices are

- upper lip—$150 per session/ $390 for a package of 3 sessions
- chin—$250 per session/ $630 for a package of 3 sessions
- full leg (thigh to ankle)—$650 per leg per session/ $910 for a package of 3 sessions per leg (and girlfriends, you do have two!)
- bikini area—$350 per session/ $910 for a package of 3 sessions

Offices usually offer discounts if you combine procedures (chin and lip), and for more than three sessions. Ask!!!

11

DERMABRASION

Have you ever used an electric sander to refinish vintage furniture? Well, the principle in dermabrasion is pretty much the same. It is an excellent way to remove acne scars, and it can even be used on patients with active acne. This can help prevent deep pitting and permanent scarring. And about 36,000 men, women, and teens chose dermabrasion to diminish scars and facial lines in 1998, according to the American Society for Aesthetic Plastic Surgery.

The success of dermabrasion depends on the skill of the person doing the procedure because exact depths are difficult to control, depending on the amount of pressure applied and the coarseness or fineness of the peripheral device (Apfelberg, 1817).

Dermabrasion can be performed in a physician's office, an outpatient surgical facility, or a hospital. You will be given both topical anesthesia and intravenous sedation. The area to be treated is sprayed with an agent to freeze the skin. Cold packs to numb the area may be applied before it is sprayed. The top layers of your skin are then "sanded" with an attachment, like a wire brush, that is on a high-speed rotary instrument (something like the dentist uses to polish your teeth). The procedure lasts from thirty to sixty minutes. There can be quite a bit of bleeding—or, should we say, *spraying* of blood!

Like laser resurfacing, your skin may be covered with Flexzan bandages, or left open to heal. Swelling is considerable. A crust, which loosens and falls off in several days, begins to form a few days after the procedure. You might be told to wash the crust with a mild soap and tap water, but *don't pick! Don't pull the crusts off!* You can cause scarring.

After the crusts fall off, the skin appears a deep pink, but it fades in three to six weeks. During this period, special soaps and cosmetics may be recommended and men are allowed to shave with mild shaving creams. You should, however, avoid medicated or scented cosmetics and hairspray on the skin.

If you are prone to acne, you will probably see an outbreak of whiteheads or little pimples (milia). Please tell your doctor, and you will be given medication to treat them. *Don't pick or squeeze!* Don't expose your skin to sunlight for several weeks, even when you walk between your house to the car. If you exercise or go to the gym, you need to stop for ten days to two weeks, and ask your physician when you can resume normal activities. For one thing, your face will swell tremendously if you exert yourself.

Complications are less common than with laser, but you can still hyperpigment (get dark blotches). If you do, your doctor can give you home treatments to even out the color of your skin. Also, don't expect perfect skin after one treatment. For acne scars, especially, you may have to repeat the procedure.

DAISY'S STORY

A pretty girl is like a melody, and Daisy—sunny, sweet, and as wholesome as the Midwest she calls home—was beauty-pageant lovely. Then in college, Daisy suddenly found herself breaking out with severe acne, a problem she never had before. Even with tetracycline, she ended up with significant scarring and a heavy heart. She never again stepped out of the house without makeup to disguise her blemished face. There was not a day when the condition of her skin didn't bother her, even after she married and had her children. "I couldn't stand it," she said. She dreamed of a smooth complexion, and avoided mirrors.

Finally, when her children got a little older and her family could afford the cost, she looked into the ways she might make her dream come true. Smart and resourceful, she did her research and decided on dermabrasion. Because she works as a teacher, she decided to do the procedure at the end of the school year, so she would have the summer months to recover. She told very few people.

She says,

I went into the procedure realistically, with the right expectations. I was hoping to see a 50 percent improvement, not perfect skin. I expected some pain and knew I would be swollen and red. The pain was far less than I anticipated, but while I had the bandages on, I avoided mirrors completely. I refused to even peek. I had the procedure on a Monday. They gave me Valium and an IV drip. I didn't feel a thing. And I had little to no pain afterward. I had the procedure on the entire area from below my eyes, right down to my chin.

On Thursday, I stood in the shower and let the bandages just fall off. Okay, I'm a wuss! But the hardest thing was looking in the mirror for the first time. Even though I had seen pictures of other people and was prepared, I looked—and cried! I was so swollen and red, I didn't even look like me. I remembered that the doctor told me it would take a full six months to see the real results. But I'm an emotional person and the tears just rolled!

"I did the research, and I felt safer with dermabrasion than laser for removing my acne scars. It was the first procedure I ever had, and I just felt more comfortable with dermabrasion."

DAISY

Also, when the bandages came off, the pain started. My face felt burning and achy. I took two Darvocet and hurt all day. After that, it was fine, and even with that one day of discomfort, the procedure was never the ordeal I expected. For three weeks it looked as if I had a terrible sunburn. Then the pink faded. I followed all instructions to the letter—I even went to the grocery store without makeup, the first time I went out in public without makeup since I was a teenager. I was determined to follow orders and take no chances. I used Bag Balm as a moisturizer, and when I did get some hyperpigmentation, I used the bleaching cream. I also did break out with milia, and since I had the procedure done in June, it was rough avoiding the sun all summer. But I did it!

When I went back to school in the fall, some people said that I must have had a great summer 'cause I looked so good.

I will definitely go back and have the procedure done again, so I can have the perfect skin of my dreams. But I look so good now, I am seriously considering entering a beauty contest again—another dream that I hope comes true!

Also—and I need to say this—doing this procedure opened my eyes. I once thought a person should be happy with the way they were, even though I wasn't. I didn't really "approve" of cosmetic surgery in my heart. In the Midwest, where I live, it's not something people do. But having the dermabrasion lifted a shadow from my life. It boosted my self-esteem tremendously. Now I understand, and feel no one should go on feeling badly about themselves when there is help.

Our Recommendations on Dermabrasion

For acne or upper-lip lines, dermabrasion is a first-choice option to consider. It works. Laser can be controlled better and actually tightens the skin, but it has a longer healing process. Balance it out. Do the research, talk to your doctor, and, like Daisy, go with the procedure that makes you feel confident and comfortable.

MICRODERMABRASION— A DERMABRASION ALTERNATIVE?

You've probably heard the buzz about the "lunchtime peel" you can get during your lunch break and go right back to the office without any downtime. Brand names include The Power Peel™, Parisian Peel™, or Derma Peel™. The technique itself is called microdermabrasion. Whatever you call it, it's a mini-sandblasting using very fine crystals (aluminum microcrystals) on your skin. Introduced in Europe a decade ago, the results look promising, but it hasn't been in use in America long enough for us to guarantee results. We can say that what we've seen is encouraging.

There are some obvious advantages. It is relatively inexpensive, has few or no side effects, and there is no "downtime" or recovery time after treatment. Skin may be slightly red for thirty minutes to six hours, but makeup can be applied immediately. There is no pain, no blood, no crusting, or need for anesthesia. In fact, it does not require a doctor to administer the treatment.

Microdermabrasion is safe for use on other parts of the body besides the face, such as the back of your hands, chest or breasts, and neck. Also, microdermabrasion is safe for darker and very dark complexions. It can be used on active acne, and to treat

- fine lines and wrinkles
- acne scars

"Right before this book went to press I had an AlloDerm implant in my upper lip and dermabrasion in the area between the nose and lip. The result was fabulous: no more little vertical wrinkles and a youthful lip line. Best of all, a new procedure to speed healing—a wet bandage that was actually stitched to my face (that sounds painful, but wasn't after all)—left my skin a light blush pink from the dermabrasion with no crusts or scabs after just three days. Susan says I have skin that responds well to dermabrasion and not all girlfriends will heal as painlessly or as fast, but I ended up with beautiful, competely smooth skin. I give this combo two thumbs up. I love the results."

CHARLEE GANNY

- stretch marks

- keloids and other scars

- enlarged or oily pores and blackheads or whiteheads

- sun-damaged skin

- age spots and other surface marks

- melasma (blotchy brown hyperpigmented patches that have an irregular shape and may be distributed over the cheeks, forehead, upper lip, and neck) on dark complexions

So what's the catch? Obviously, this is a very light peel, and you might require several treatments to get significant results. Susan has had it done. Charlee says she feels it is effective as a chemical peel, and the experience is much more pleasant. It improved her skin texture and appearance, although only temporarily. As part of getting ready for a special event, she says the light dermabrasion is a must!

The only caution we offer is to remember: When something sounds too good to be true, it usually is.

12

THE MIRACLES OF CHEMISTRY

Let's talk chemical peels. First there was Phenol. Phyllis Diller had it along with her famous face-lift, and her skin looked fantastic. Yes, it is true. This granddaddy of all chemical peels does a great job—if you don't die, can stand the excruciating pain, and don't mind having your skin "depigmented"—in other words, it turns white. Let's not be flip about this. *Phenol is dangerous. Don't do it.*

Any chemical peel is a controlled wounding or burning of the skin. The physician decides on the depth of the wounding, based on how much sun damage has occurred. As the new skin forms, the surface of the skin may appear years younger. Only in deep peels is there some shrinkage of the underlying collagen to tighten the skin.

Chemical peels done in the doctor's office can help with acne scarring, freckles, age spots, and melasma (dark spots which are often found in women who are pregnant or taking birth-control pills). Pre-cancerous conditions such as keratoses (thick, rough, reddish growths) also respond well to chemical peels.

There are many types of safe chemical peels, but the type most often administered in a surgical facility or hospital is a trichloroacetic acid (TCA) peel or a combination of TCA and an alpha-hydroxy acid (AHA) peel. These TCA peels can alter the skin's surface structurally much in the same way as risky phenol peels and dermabrasion (editorial, 316). Like all kinds of chemical peels, the difficulty of controlling the depth of the peel remains, and there are complications such as hyperpigmentation and hypertrophic scarring. Downtime can be about the same as a dermabrasion, with crusting, peeling, and redness. In truth, TCA peels have pretty much been replaced by laser. But TCA peels are still an option for resurfacing the skin and removing wrinkles.

Do peels hurt? Yes, and the deeper the peel, the more it hurts or burns. Chemical peels are, after all, a "wounding" of the skin. It is not easy to lie there with chemicals eating into your skin, feeling the air of the fan that is set up during the duration of the peel to cool the burning sensation. The procedure can last from twenty minutes to one hour or more. Afterward, you might be bandaged for a day or two. Swelling is expected, and you will probably be advised to keep your head elevated.

As the skin heals, crusts begin to form, and some tingling and itching may occur. Cool compresses can reduce these sensations. After the crusts fall off, the skin is bright pink, which gradually fades over the next few weeks. Maximum improvement of damaged skin ranges from 75 to 85 percent and most women view the results as dramatic.

STILL ANOTHER ACNE HEARTBREAK—ICE-PICK SCARS

Ice-pick scars may be superficial or deep, and most often appear on the cheeks. The surface of the scar is fairly small with a jagged edge, sharp margins, and steep sides. But as the scar goes deeper into the skin, it widens under the surface. Ice-pick scars *do not* respond favorably to chemical peels. Deeper peels might even make the scar appear larger, as the wider, deeper scar levels are exposed. The best way to remove this type of acne scar is using a "punch excision," which is a procedure that removes the scarred area and replaces the plug with skin from another area of the body. Later this replaced skin can be dermabraded to match the level of the rest of the face if needed.

An alternative to a deep peel is a salon-administered, light alpha-hydroxy acid peel. (There are five kinds of fruit acids. The one with the smallest molecule is glycolic acid. It is a superb resurfacing agent.) While these peels produce little real change in the structure of the skin, repeated superficial peels can gradually reduce the appearance of acne, melasma, and some types of scars (Duffy, 181). A salon peel is generally a very safe and pleasant element in a good facial. It will smooth finer wrinkles and enhance the absorption of moisturizers. Also, by improving hydration it will "plump up" your skin so it looks firmer or "filled out." This will also reduce the appearance of the size of your pores. Light peels, by plumping up the skin, will improve the overall appearance of pore size. Salon peels will help maintain your skin's youthful appearance, and you'll feel wonderfully pampered; so peels can be as good for the spirit as for the flesh. Do it regularly if you can afford it, or have one occasionally for a special treat.

AT-HOME TREATMENTS

Although you will not get the dramatic results of a surgical procedure from an at-home treatment, you can do a great deal to improve the visual appearance of your skin, including the texture. To give you a quick overview, glycolic products resurface your skin and plump it up; they may even promote the formation of collagen, especially when combined with vitamin C. Glycolic acid plus salicylic acid and benzoyl-peroxide products can significantly heal and prevent acne without the use of antibiotics. You can fade blotchiness with bleaching agents. And you can diminish fine lines and even reverse sun damage with Retin-A.

Glycolic Products

Alpha-hydroxy acid products are abundant at the cosmetics counter or even in the supermarket. They are not, however, equally effective.

> **REMINDER**
>
> **A**s with all types of skin resurfacing, any woman using Accutane should not have a peel, not even one from a salon.

What should you look for? First of all, you want to use a facial wash, night cream, or day moisturizer that contains glycolic acid, the most effective of the alpha-hydroxy acids. Second, you want it in a strong-enough concentration to do some good—and since strengths aren't listed, you may have to go by trial and error (or price: good glycolic products will cost $30 and up).

Which product lines are best? There are dozens of excellent ones. However, ask your dermatologist or plastic surgeon for a recommendation; many have their own formulas. The OBAGI® skin care system, for example, has several products that are stronger than over-the-counter formulas and can only be obtained through a physician. With OBAGI, wrinkle reduction and improvement in overall skin quality is often spectacular, particularly with OBAGI's new patented Blue Peel, a chemical peel. Because the Blue Peel allows the provider to precisely control the depth of the peel, it has gotten great results, even for dark complexions and brown skin!

The over-the-counter products Susan and Charlee both use for daily skin care are made by Jan Marini Skin Research Inc. Try Jan Marini's Bioclear Cream if you are prone to pimples or blackheads. It is fantastic! And Jan Marini's C-Esta™ Lips is a wonderful "plumper-upper" and softener to put on under lipstick. Jan Marini has a toll free number (1-800-347-2223) that you can call. Be advised, that a good product is relatively expensive.

One advance in skin-care products are those that try to deliver vitamin C topically to your skin. Skin is very vulnerable to vitamin C deficiency, and any time of stress—emotional or physical—can deplete your skin's supply. If you are under chronic stress, your skin shows it. But it is very difficult to get vitamin C to the skin topically because vitamin C loses its potency when exposed to sun or heat. Also, it is difficult to deliver it to the deeper levels of skin. There are products on the market that claim to do this—with varying levels of success. Jan Marini's C-Esta line, mentioned earlier, is one of them. Some women swear by the C–Esta products, and they're definitely worth a try.

Anti-acne Products

Happily, one line of products that definitely work are those developed to heal or prevent acne breakouts. Products which combine glycolic acid with salicylic acid do a superior job of removing the cells that block the follicle (blocked follicles allow the acne bacteria, "P–acne bacteria," to thrive). Salicylic acid is endorsed by the American Academy of Dermatology as an agent that retards or reverses the formation of comedones. These are small, firm whitish bumps under the skin that become acne lesions. An open comedone is what you call a "blackhead."

THE BLACKHEAD DILEMMA

When blackheads are squeezed, only the contents in the opening of the pore are eliminated and matter from this pore (called a pilosebaceous follicle) pushes forward and reappears in a few hours. Astringents, masks, scrubs, extractions, and those popular nose strips have only a temporary effect, and do nothing to interrupt the acne process. Your best bet is to use a combination glycolic- and salicylic-acid product that gets at the source of the problem.

Benzoyl peroxide, a powerful antibacterial agent, is endorsed by the American Academy of Dermatology as effective in acne therapy. It rapidly destroys P–acne bacteria, as well as yeast and other organisms. The bacteria does not develop a resistance to benzoyl peroxide, even after years of continuous use. It is extremely safe. It will help clear acne lesions and prevent breakouts. Products, however, should be applied to the entire area affected by acne, not just to individual lesions. But if you develop a serious acne problem, get professional help immediately to avoid scarring. Don't suffer!

Tretinoin, or Retin-A

Girlfriends, very few products work. This one does. It honest-to-God removes wrinkles—not the *appearance* of wrinkles; it sends the damn things packing. So why aren't you using it? If you are over thirty-five, you should be. It's never too late to start; you will see improvement even if you are over eighty. If you still have blemishes, Retin-A will control your acne, too.

Retin-A makes skin appear smoother, thicker, and fuller. When examined under a microscope, this "new" skin resembles that of a young child. It has more protein, skin cells, and blood vessels, which provide many of the needed nutrients to the skin surface. Fine wrinkles soften, certain discolorations lighten or completely disappear, and some pre-cancerous conditions are eradicated. In fact, some doctors think that Retin-A can prevent the development of certain skin cancers. Plus, its cost is close to the price of the pink, anti-wrinkle "Promises in a Jar" from the cosmetics counter. Okay, so it's not prettied-up in a fancy package; it's just in a metal tube with a prescription label stuck on it. The stuff works. Pretty terrific!

Non-prescription versions of Retin-A are on the market, and they may work to some degree. Jan Marini carries a vitamin-A line developed by Dr. James Fulton, the same doctor who helped develop Retin-A. It is called Factor-A®, and it is patented. It promises to lessen the side effects of Retin-A by 80 percent—but does it work as well? It definitely improves the appearance of the skin, but does it change the underlying structure? The jury is still out on that.

There's always a tradeoff!

As good as the new products are in helping keep your skin youthful, there is a negative you may not know about. Here it is:

> Virtually all the techniques we now use to increase the
> youthful appearance of the skin (i.e., glycolic peels,

trichloroacetic acid peels, and topical tretinoin) create increased epidermal translucency that allows the underlying telangiectasia and vascularity to show through [seeing the redness of capillaries and veins near the surface of the skin—in other words, a rash on your cheeks and a red nose]. Patients will often recognize correctly that their skin is more youthful, but the telangiectasia and vascularity are more pronounced. This is especially apparent with people undergoing CO2 laser resurfacing and those who use topical tretinoin [Retin-A] chronically (Mayl, 164, 166).

If you have fragile skin and tend to get a redness on your cheeks, for instance, you should avoid the use of buff puffs and abrasive washes. PABA-containing sunscreens can also be irritating; choose one without PABA (Mayl, page 164).

BOTOX

The one thing that laser just doesn't do well is remove dynamic wrinkles, the ones caused by facial movement. Now there is good news and bad news. The good news is that Botox works better than you can imagine to eliminate wrinkles caused by movement (like frown lines between your eyes). The bad news is that it doesn't work for long, especially the first time you get an injection.

Botox is a relatively new procedure that uses botulinum toxin to weaken or paralyze the facial muscles beneath the skin that create expression lines, such as worry and frown lines, crow's-feet, laugh lines, and other dynamic wrinkles. It is the fastest-growing plastic surgery procedure, jumping from 65,157 in 1997, to 157,439 procedures performed in 1998—an increase of 142 percent!

Botox is injected into various locations of the face. The needle is extremely small and doesn't cause severe pain, but it will cause discomfort. If you've had collagen or fat injections, it's very

---

THE CHEAPEST AND BEST MOISTURIZER— WATER

If you want to see plumper, fuller skin, drink *at least* 8 glasses of water a day. Few of us do. And we drink caffeine—which further dehydrates us. But if you make the effort, you will see visible results—and more youthful-looking skin.

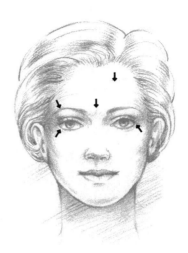

Botox injections

similar. It really doesn't hurt much, but you certainly will feel twinges and tingles.

Depending on how many places on the face you are having injected, the procedure can last from between ten and thirty minutes. Because there is no sedative or anesthetic used, you can hop right up off the table or out of the chair and go about your normal routine. Sometimes you will be told not to lie down for three or four hours after treatment. It actually takes three to five days before you see the full effects of the procedure. The results can be miraculous—the wrinkles vanish.

When the toxin begins to wear off, the wrinkles slowly come back; however, they may not appear as deep. It usually takes two or three injections to keep a smooth, youthful appearance over the course of a year. As the standard cover-your-ass phrase says: "Results vary widely."

A side effect might be some bruising at the injection site. Another that occurs only rarely is a slight drooping of the eyebrow or upper eyelid. Fortunately, when this occurs, it goes away on its own in two to three weeks. Teresa had a strange, and perhaps unique reaction: She lost her ability to smile with her upper lip for about a month. Can your whole face get paralyzed? That's a common question and concern. The answer is no. Can the botulism toxin poison you? Again, in the hands of an experienced doctor, the answer is no. (But you can only use a certain amount; an overdose *could* poison you.)

Actually, the product is terrific. Unfortunately Botox is quite expensive. Three treatments that may or may not last, will cost you well over a thousand dollars. However, Botox is a good option if you don't want a brow-lift. It's wonderful if you have a big event coming up . . . like your wedding (see Teresa's story below). Even with the drawbacks, it is still better than two "fillers," collagen and fat injections.

COLLAGEN INJECTIONS, FAT INJECTIONS, AND ALLODERM

Bossy's Gift to Your Face

It is made from cows, and it ends up pumped into your face. In 1998 367,170 people, mostly women, had collagen injections (American Society for Aesthetic Plastic Surgery). But that number is dropping. Collagen held so much promise once upon a time; it seemed like a great leap forward, a safe way to fill up the indentations in your face caused by wrinkles or blemishes. It could even give you great lips! Sure, you had to get a skin test first to make sure you weren't allergic to this extract made from cows . . . and no, you couldn't be squeamish about getting a needle in your face. But other than that, it was quick and easy—and instantly satisfying. At least, it was satisfying for a fleeting instant.

Amid the hype and hope of collagen's introduction for use in plastic surgery, we were promised that collagen injections would last for months. Charlee's first injection of collagen lasted seventy-two hours. She immediately phoned for a "touch-up" appointment. Of course, the touch-up shot was for a price. She thought she was just unlucky that her body had reabsorbed the collagen with such great efficiency. Later, she discovered that many women experience collagen as a brief, bittersweet experience.

Actually collagen is still an option for two reasons. First of all, you can use it for temporary wrinkle removal for a big event. Go ahead and schedule your injection a few days before your hair and nail appointments, and the initial swelling will be gone in time. Second, if you are thinking of using AlloDerm to plump up your top lip or to fill in your nasolabial folds (the lines from your nose and to the edges of your mouth), you can see what the final results will look like by using collagen or fat injections before taking the more expensive route.

Are there any other complications with collagen? Yes, but they are rare. Charlee once got an infection at the injection site (from putting on makeup). People can be allergic to the material. An inexperienced practitioner can create a disaster by injecting it in the wrong place—or even create an embolism. But again, these serious complications are very unusual.

Your Butt's Gift to Your Face

The next great leap forward in trying to fill up wrinkles was to move your own fat from one part of your body (usually your buttocks) to another. It has never been as popular as collagen, although 73,419 Americans underwent the procedure in 1998 (American Society for Aesthetic Plastic Surgery). Using the same technology as liposuction, fat is extracted, processed, and injected into your frown lines, your nasolabial folds, or even your lips. Because it's your own fat, your body can't reject it. Theoretically, it lasts longer and isn't completely reabsorbed by your body, leaving the wrinkles diminished.

Fat injections are a better option that collagen as far as rejection goes. If they are filling a wrinkle that is not a dynamic wrinkle (from muscular movement), they do last longer. But the downside is that the extraction of the fat from your buttock can leave a depression.

So as a temporary remedy for wrinkles, or as a preview of what a permanent solution might look like, fat injections have their place . . . and leave their mark.

AlloDerm

When it comes to wrinkle fillers, AlloDerm is the latest option. It is long-lasting; your body accepts it without rejection, and it does a fantastic job. So what's the problem? Well . . .

First of all, AlloDerm is made from real human skin—not yours. So, whose skin is it? Yep, you guessed it, an organ donor's (skin is an organ, your body's largest). The human donor's skin is processed so that all the cells of the epidermis and dermis are removed; only the protein framework is left; it has no human cells, and it is freeze-dried.

Is AlloDerm safe? Rigorous donor screening has made transplanted grafts very safe from HIV or other diseases. In addition, the tissue is processed to kill any viral matter, including HIV. Over the last ten years, more than one million tissue grafts have been safely transplanted. It is especially effective when used with Botox for dynamic wrinkles.

AlloDerm must be put in place surgically; it is not injected. Once in your body, your own tissue grows around it.

TERESA'S STORY

It was a whirlwind romance. He was getting married for the first time, at age thirty-eight. Teresa, now forty, had been married, briefly, in her twenties, but this time she was seeing rainbows. Both the bride and groom wanted a big wedding, with the bride wearing white and a whole host of bridesmaids in chic, elegant black.

At the first chic, pricey bridal salon that Teresa entered after calling for an appointment, she was greeted by a smiling, effusive saleswoman who said, gushing, "And where's the bride?" "I'm the bride," a crushed Teresa murmured.

"The woman didn't know where to look," Teresa remembers. Actually, Teresa looks at least ten years younger than her age . . . now. Back then, she had the deepest, most noticeable frown lines known to woman between her eyes. They not only added years to her face, "they made me look as if I were projecting an emotion I wasn't feeling—unhappiness or worry. I thought about getting Botox and AlloDerm implants before my wedding, but chickened out, thinking, 'What if something goes wrong?' What went wrong is that I have three hundred professionally taken, expensive wedding photos—of me frowning."

Teresa's first Botox injection lasted about three months; her second, nearly a year; and then she had a third injection and Allo-Derm implants.

I did have two incisions below my eyebrows, and two black eyes! I had to go back to work, and I didn't know what to tell people. I finally wore sunglasses and said I was in a minor car accident, but that the sunglasses got pushed into my nose—and gave me swelling and two black eyes.

The excuse worked perfectly. No one suspected a thing, though I had a bad moment when a coworker asked me a few weeks later if I had gotten my car fixed yet . . . and I didn't know what she was talking about.

I no longer look like a perpetual grump. I love it!

NOW WHAT DO I DO?

13

FINDING A DOCTOR

Okay, you're interested in plastic surgery. You're *really* interested. Now, how do you take the most important step of all—finding the right plastic surgeon for you?

One resource we looked at said there is no "infallible method" for choosing a plastic surgeon or guaranteeing a good result (*Sun-Sentinel,* December 5, 1998). We beg to differ. You can choose a wonderful plastic surgeon. No one can guarantee 100 percent good results, but we think you deserve a "limited warranty" that covers the skill of the doctor, your preparation for surgery, the quality of the equipment and staff, and your post-op care. So we want a 99 percent guarantee of good results that only an act of God or a hidden medical condition can void.

Okay, so we're picky. You need to be, too.

First we're going to tell you the basics—the steps you must take, no matter where you are or whom you decide to see. This is your homework. Failing this assignment can be deadly.

Then we're going to tell you some other things to do that we know, from insider experience and from our girlfriends.

Finally, we are going to help you out with some essentials of what to do and say during your consultation with the surgeon—

including our strong preference for the use of a girlfriend advocate. So here goes. . . .

First You Need a Name

How do you find a surgeon—a *good* surgeon? You need names. Where do you get them?

- Referrals from the accrediting board (see the sidebar on www.plasticsurgery.org in this chapter). If you want to stay in your area, you can get the names of all the board-certified surgeons within easy traveling distance of your location. Those names can be a checklist to work from.

- Patients. If you know someone who has had plastic surgery with good results, get the name of her doctor. But, listen carefully: Many women go to a doctor because a friend, or even just an acquaintance, said, "This doctor is really good"; they never check further. *Please, don't take anyone's word to judge a doctor's worth.* Use the recommendation as a starting point only!

- Surgical nurses. A friend, a friend of a friend, a relative . . . someone you know is a nurse. If she isn't an operating-room nurse, she'll know one. Nurses will give it to you straight. They'll not only give you names; they'll let you know whom to trust. They've seen the doctor at work. Ask the nurse which doctor she would choose if she were having the particular surgery you are considering. Then put a *big* star next to that name. Nurses are insiders—and the best judge of doctors we know.

  Speaking of the opinions of nurses, what about others in the medical profession? Should you ask your family doctor or gynecologist for a referral? If you have a close friend who is a doctor, sure, go ahead and ask. If you have a close relative who is a doctor, go ahead and ask. But other doctors . . . nope!

They'll send you to their friends, a business associate, or the guy they want to start playing golf with. If the doctor doesn't care about you as more than a patient, don't ask him or her for a name.

- Advertising. Girlfriends, first of all remember: *Caveat emptor* (Let the buyer beware)—but this is *not* a bad way to find a doctor. There's nothing wrong with getting a name from the yellow pages, the local coupon clipper, or a TV spot. Just use your common sense. The best doctors advertise. So do some bad ones. It's perfectly okay to use an ad to get a name for your list. But it's only the first step of your hunt.

Once you have your name or names, it's on to the next step.

FOLLOWING THE PAPER TRAIL

Girlfriends, put on your detective hats because you're going to do some sleuthing just like the professional private eyes do.

- Check the credentials of your doctor. You need to know the shocking truth: *There are no laws prohibiting any physician from performing a plastic-surgery procedure—even if he's never done more than take a one-day course in using the brand-new laser machine he just bought.*

Now, pay attention, girlfriends, here's the poop: *There is no medical specialty called "cosmetic surgery."* No doctor can be certified in cosmetic surgery. The specialty is called "plastic and reconstructive surgery." So here's the red flag to watch for: If a doctor calls himself a "cosmetic surgeon" or advertises "practice limited to cosmetic surgery," be suspicious—until you see the magic words, "Certified by the American Board of Plastic Surgery." Unless you see that, the doctor could be a general practitioner with little or no formal training in plastic surgery and with no board certification. Keep in mind the old joke:

Q: "What do they call a medical student who graduates last in his class?"

A: "Doctor."

You must find out specifically: Is the doctor board-certified by the American Board of Plastic Surgery (ABPS)? ABPS can be reached at (215) 587-9322. The words "board-certified" alone, aren't good enough. What if the doctor is board-certified in psychiatry and decided to go out and buy a laser machine?

Want to know the easiest way to find out if a doctor is board-certified . . . and avoid a toll call? Use your computer (or ask a friend if you are still a technophobe) and go on-line and find www.plasticsurgery.org. This is the Internet site of the American Society of Plastic Surgery. Ninety-seven percent of all physicians certified by the American Board of Plastic Surgery are members. You can also call the Society at 1-800-635-0635. It's a great way to start.

Are any other doctors besides board-certified plastic surgeons qualified to perform a specific "aesthetic" plastic-surgery procedure? Maybe. A board-certified dermatologist may do a good job of skin resurfacing with lasers, dermabrasion, or chemical peels. An otolaryngologist (head and neck specialist) might do a superb septoplasty (repair of the inside of the nose). An ophthalmologist can do a blepharoplasty on your eyelids. However, if you are having surgery to improve your appearance—not a medical condition—a board-certified plastic surgeon is going to be most experienced in the aesthetics of the profession.

• Check out lawsuits against a doctor. A malpractice suit against a doctor is not unusual, nor does it mean he is a bad doctor—*unless* there are three medical malpractice suits against a doctor within five years. That's a warning sign that there are problems.

How do you know if a doctor is in legal trouble? Some states make it easy to find out.

In Florida, you can check with the Florida Department of Insurance (www.doi.state.fl.us) to see if a doctor has settled any claims, and you can contact the Florida Agency for Health Care Administration (1-888-419-3456, or www.fdhc.state.fl.us) to see if disciplinary action has been taken against this practitioner.

In New York State, you can look at www.nysed.gov/home/regents.html to see if a doctor is licensed. You can also call the New York State Department of Health at 1-800-663-6114.

In other states, you have to hunt for the information by computer, by phone, or by foot. You can try calling your state agencies and the local American Medical Association office, or you can personally go to your county courthouse to see if a suit has been filed in your area (sorry, but you can't get this information by phone).

- Check to see if the surgeon has privileges to perform the procedure you are considering at *an accredited hospital* in your community—even if the procedure is going to be performed in the doctor's own surgical facility. In other words, is Dr. X permitted to perform tummy tucks at General Hospital? Don't take anyone's word for it—call that hospital to verify that this is so. If the doctor's privileges are suspended or don't exist, *run*, don't walk, to the nearest exit.

- Check out the certification of the doctor's own surgical facility. It is less expensive and, quite frankly, often safer to have your surgery done in the doctor's own facility. There are several good reasons. In a private facility, you will be exposed to far less risk of infection or of catching someone else's disease (after all, there aren't any sick people here). You receive one-on-one attention and compassion; the staff cares about keeping you happy. Your money, not an insurance company's, is paying their salary.

WWW.PLASTIC SURGERY.ORG

Not all Internet sites give you information you can rely on. This one does. It is user-friendly. It provides a profile of the specific doctor you are considering or offers you referrals to several doctors in your area. You can also get information on the specific procedure you are considering. Take the time to investigate this. It's an invaluable research tool.

Moreover, in a good facility, the equipment is often better than in a hospital. So how do you know if a facility is top-notch?

It's easy if the office is accredited, but right now (this may change by the time you read this) only California, Nevada, Maryland, and Georgia *require* accreditation of office surgical facilities. Legislation specifically directed toward ensuring consumer protection and quality in office-based practices has been passed in California, Florida, and New Jersey, and is pending in New York (Joas, 301). Doctors in other states, anticipating that someday all states may require accreditation, have begun getting accreditation on their own.

There are two primary accrediting agencies:

AAAHC (Accreditation Association for Ambulatory Health Care, Inc.)
9933 Lawler Ave
Skokie, IL 60077-3708
Tel: (847) 676-9610
Fax: (847) 676-9628

AAAASF (American Association for Accreditation of Ambulatory Surgery Facilities)
102 Allanson Road
Mundelein, IL 60060
Tel: (847) 949-6058
Fax: (847) 566-4580

So, your first step is to ask about office accreditation. Is the office accredited? If the office is *not* accredited, you can ask how it is equipped, then contact one of the agencies above to see if the facility meets their standards. If not, cross it off your list.

• Check the credentials of the person administering the anesthesia. He or she should either be a "certified registered nurse anesthetist" or a "physician anesthesiologist." Find out!

Going Beyond the Paper Trail

Okay, all the basics check out. Now you need to find a surgeon whom you like and who inspires confidence. Most of all, you need someone who does beautiful work with his or her hands. A doctor can be academically brilliant but not a great surgeon. You need to see your doctor in action and view the results of his or her handiwork.

Here is what we suggest:

Go in for a consultation. We'll give you some questions to ask below. But beyond words, you will need to do the following.

- See the doctor's portfolio of the procedure or procedures you are interested in. This will be a collection of "before" and "after" photos of the patients he or she has operated on. Look it over carefully. Look for patients with a condition or body type similar to yours. Keep in mind, this is the doctor's *best* work.

- Ask if any of the doctor's staff has had plastic surgery from the doctor. If the doctor is good, many of his or her staff people will have had procedures done. Ask to talk to them about their procedures. The fact that people who work in the office have been operated on by the doctor is a good sign. If the office or nursing staff hasn't gotten any plastic surgery, you need to wonder why not.

- Ask to talk to some of the doctor's patients who are similar to you and had the same kind of surgery. Remember, the doctor cannot give you anyone's name because of patient confidentiality. What he or she *can* do is to give your name to a patient who can call you. So you have to be willing (and sign a consent form) to have *your* name given to someone else. Usually, a good doctor will have patients who are open and eager to share their good experience and great results with you.

Going In for a Consultation

Attention, girlfriends: *You have to pay for a consultation.* Find out how much the doctor charges *before* you make an appointment. Fees can range from $50 to a few hundred dollars. Call several doctors to find out what most surgeons charge in your area of the country.

Taking Along a Friend-Advocate

After you make the appointment, we recommend you do not go alone. Our first choice for a companion is a friend-advocate. A friend-advocate is a friend or family member *who is supportive* of your decision to have plastic surgery—*not* someone who is skeptical or hostile. The job of the friend-advocate is to write down what the surgeon says. Your job is to ask questions and listen to answers. You can also allow the friend-advocate to ask a question, if she wishes, but not more than one or two. *You* do the talking, not the friend-advocate. Make this clear ahead of time! Discuss it. Don't leave it to chance.

After the consultation, the friend-advocate should hand over to you the notes she took. Later—and probably at a later time than the car ride home—you should discuss the consultation with the friend-advocate. Don't ask, "What do you think?" Ask the friend-advocate specific questions, whose answers will be based on direct observations and facts. Here are some examples:

- "Did the doctor give a clear answer when I asked about the risks of the procedure?"
- "Was the staff professional and courteous when you observed them?"
- "Would you say the atmosphere was friendly? Why or why not?"
- "Did you react negatively to any aspect of the consultation?"

- "What would you say were the most positive things about this plastic surgeon?"

Get the idea? Ask your friend-advocate direct questions that require reasoned answers. Decide whether you agree or disagree. *Do not ask your friend-advocate, "What should I do?" That is your decision, and yours alone.*

Why not take a spouse or a significant other? Of course, you can. But . . . ! Sometimes the person you love isn't the best person to have along when you are making a decision about yourself. He's a great person to take you in for the procedure, to wait and worry during the operation, and to be there when it's over and lovingly take you home. Yet in these early stages, in the decision-making process, you need to be in control. Chances are he has mixed feelings about your wanting surgery, and, in fact, he might even be dead set against it out of concern for your safety. And let's be honest here: He might be against it because of the cost.

Okay, you have someone to accompany you to the consultation. Here's the next step.

CHARLEE'S FAIL-SAFE METHOD

A consultation is revealing, but it is only an interview. I have another suggestion. If you like what you have found by following your paper trail, or if you've heard good things about a surgeon, consider actually having a small procedure done. Make it one that will cost you under $500. For instance, if you need a mole removed [probably covered by insurance], or if you would like a Botox, fat, or collagen injection for a special event, go in for a consultation about it. If you like what you hear, go in for the procedure. By taking this first step before diving in for major surgery, you will have the opportunity to sit in the waiting room with other patients, and you can start talking to them. You will get to experience the surgeon's work. You will get to know the staff and feel the ambience of the office—only if I had a successful experience, was impressed by the doctor, and established a rapport with the doctor and staff, would I go back to have a major procedure. That's what I did, and no, I didn't choose the first plastic surgeon I went to. But I did choose the best.

What to Tell and What to Ask During the Consultation

Opening the interview.

Begin by telling the surgeon, as specifically as possible, what part of your body you are concerned about, and what you'd like as a result. Some examples:

- "I feel my buttocks and thighs are out of proportion with the rest of my body. I would like to go from my present size to about two clothing sizes smaller, and have a better contour—not this bulge on my outer thigh. What do you recommend?"

- "I have fat legs and ankles. I'd like to look better when I wear a dress and not have to cover them up. Can I get a thinner look? How much thinner?"

- "I have loose skin on my stomach. What can you do?"

- "I want to get rid of the wrinkles around my eyes."

- "I have acne scars. Can I get rid of them? What can you do?"

Listen closely to his or her answer to your initial question. Be sure that the following information is provided by the doctor's answers. If not, be sure to ask,

- Is this the only procedure he or she recommends for the problem?

- What are the pros and cons of the procedure recommended?

- Do you have any other options?

- Can you see photos of the doctor's results with this procedure? (Remember, you might not get the same results.)

But what if the doctor takes you over to a computer, and says, "Let me show you what we can do." *Pass. Don't do it.* Say you'd rather talk to him or her instead. Here's why. . . .

Should your consultation include computer imaging?

Sorry, but Susan doesn't recommend it—and she should know! The computer image of what you would look like after the operation has no basis in reality. That reality is your flesh and blood. A computer picture provides no guarantee of results. In fact, it may set up false or unrealistic expectations—because what it shows you is the ideal, and not usually what can be accomplished in real life.

Instead, let the physician explain, very carefully, what he or she can do and what results can be expected. Look at examples of the surgeon's work in the portfolio or on a real patient. Also, be able to describe as clearly as possible what results you want—and be sure to ask how closely the surgeon feels he can come to meeting your expectations. Realize you may have to lower your expectations; what you want may be impossible to attain.

Second-round questions.

Next, ask when the doctor last performed this operation. Ask how many of these procedures the doctor has performed in the past year.

You might also ask what procedure your doctor performs most often. In other words, he may do a fabulous face-lift and be known for them, but doesn't do well with liposuction. You should feel comfortable that the surgeon is well-experienced and up-to-date in the procedure you're considering.

Give him the third degree.

Finally, and of critical importance, ask what complications the doctor has had for this procedure. *Every* doctor experiences complications. There is nothing wrong with that; your body is not a machine; it is living tissue and tremendously complex. However, if the doctor says, "None," you know he or she is either lying or not operating frequently enough.

Then you need to ask, If there *are* complications, can the surgeon handle the problem, or does the patient get sent to see someone else?

A good surgeon can deal with a procedure's complications. However, there are *always* exceptions. For example, if a tear duct doesn't work after blepharoplasty, you will probably be sent to an ophthalmologist. But for all routine and usual complications, you want a doctor who can fix it.

ASPS Recommendations for Your Consultation (from *www.plasticsurgery.org*)

- The surgeon should answer all of your questions thoroughly, in language you can understand.

- He/she should ask about your motivations and expectations, discuss them with you, and solicit your reaction to his/her recommendations.

- He/she should offer alternatives, where appropriate, without pressuring you to consider unnecessary procedures.

- He/she should welcome questions about professional qualifications, experience, costs, and payment policies.

- He/she should make clear not only the risks of surgery, but the possible variations in outcome. If the surgeon shows you photographs of other patients, or uses computer imaging to show you possible results, it should be made clear that there is no guarantee that your results will match these.

- He/she should make sure the final decision is yours.

What it all boils down to.

- You must spend time with the surgeon before you make any decisions.

- You must like and respect the surgeon.

- You must feel comfortable and confident with him or her.

- You must listen to your gut instinct—if something inside says *no*, the decision is *no*.

- You must go slowly. Don't rush into anything. Don't make an on-the-spot decision.

- You must feel safe and cared-for in the surgical setting.

All things being equal . . .

- You will need pre- and post-operative photographs. Some doctors will make you see a photographer at a different location and have photos taken at your own expense. Others take them in the office—at no extra expense. Which is the better deal? You got it!

- Compare costs. You are not bargain-shopping, but there is no reason to be overcharged, either.

- If a compression garment or surgical bra is needed after surgery, is the price included in the surgery? Do you get one or two?

- What medication or topical applications are needed before and after surgery? Are any of them provided by the surgeon's office or are all the costs out of your pocket—in addition to the procedure's cost?

- Do you need to stay overnight at a non-hospital facility? What is it like? Who will stay with you? What does it cost?

- If any corrections are needed after the surgery, what are the fees? Are there any corrections that will be done without cost to you? Is there a discount if additional work is needed? Remember, *there is no such thing as "a little touch-up."* Any additional surgery has considerable expenses attached.

- How easy is it to get an appointment?

- How long do you have to wait in the waiting room?

- When you are shown to an examining room, how long do you have to wait?

- How does the staff treat you?

- And now, the biggie: *How easy is it to get to speak to the doctor him/herself on the phone?* If you have a problem after surgery, you don't want to be shuttled around from answering service to nurse to receptionist . . . only to wait hours, or days, for a return call.

Take the time to do your homework! By discovering all you can about your procedure and a surgeon's competency, you are taking control of your own destiny and not leaving your future to whim or to chance.

FINDING THE MONEY

The couple was young. The wife sat perched on the edge of her chair on the other side of Susan's desk, her husband in the chair next to her. Her tense body leaned slightly forward; one of her small hands was held tightly in her husband's big one. Although her face was pretty and unlined, her body, she explained in an urgent voice, had been "ravaged" by having children. Her breasts drooped, her stomach was flaccid and sagging, she had developed protruding "shelves" of fat on top of her hips below her waistline, and her once-tight butt had spread . . . and spread. When she looked in the mirror, she cried. She wanted Susan to understand that she didn't regret having her children, but between the stretch marks, the fat, and the flab, she was miserable—twenty-four hours a day.

With tears spilling down her cheeks, she told Susan that she was only thirty-one, but her body looked fifty. She wanted it fixed. The doctor had said he could do it. Now she had to have the surgeries, she explained. She just had to.

With a sinking heart, Susan figured out the costs for all the procedures—liposuction, a tummy tuck, breast uplift and augmentation, and a thighplasty. Even by doing many of the procedures at the same time to save on anesthesia and operating-room costs, the total was large—*major* money. For a struggling young family where the breadwinner was a car mechanic on salary, Susan feared the price would make the surgery impossible. Certainly they could never afford all of it . . . and maybe not any of it. When Susan gently suggested perhaps doing only one of the procedures, the wife was adamant. She needed the whole package.

Susan dreaded giving the bottom line to the eager, hopeful people across from her. But as she broke the news, she didn't see anything but smiles. What was going on?

Love.

When the young man looked at his wife, he saw how unhappy she was. She had given him children and sacrificed her youthful body—and he loved her. So he was making a sacrifice to pay for the surgery she so desperately wanted.

He was selling his Harley.

PAYING THE PRICE

How much does surgery cost? There is no simple answer. The first year for which a nationally recognized agency, the American Society for Aesthetic Plastic Surgery (ASAPS), compiled statistics was 1997. Their statistics are only for physicians'/surgeons' fees. They *do not* include fees for the surgical facility, anesthesia, medical tests, prescriptions, surgical garments, or other miscellaneous costs related to surgery. Why? These costs have no standard fee. They vary with your individual needs, your geographical location, and where your surgery is performed—either a hospital, or a physician's office or facility. They may range from as "little" as a thousand dollars, to several thousand dollars. These costs can be also be reduced if you have more than one procedure at a time; for example, if you have laser resurfacing and a face-lift at the same time, or a nose job and breast augmentation at the same time. *You must ask:* What are the average *total* costs in your doctor's office for the procedure or procedures you are considering?

Following is the 1998 range of physician/surgeon fees per procedure from the ASAPS (see page 240). Remember "per procedure" means just that—if you want liposuction on your thighs *and* your hips, that is *two* procedures; if you want a fat injection in your nasolabial folds *and* your frown lines, that is *two* procedures. Each surgery site counts as a separate procedure.

"Show Me the Money!"

When you opt for cosmetic surgery, you have to pay "up front." It's the rule. "No tickee, no surgery." Before you go under the knife, the bill must be paid *in full*—except for the procedures your insurance will cover. (We'll give you an overview of insurance help below.) Also . . .

- Be aware that you will have to pay more if you want "touch-ups" or changes after the surgery.

- Be aware that you will have medication costs and some costs for post-op supplies (see chapter 15, "Preparing Mentally and Physically for Surgery").

- Be aware that there may be pre-admission testing and blood-work costs.

- Be aware that you may have hidden costs, such as cab fare, grocery delivery, babysitters, caregivers, or take-out food for your husband and/or kids.

- Be aware that you will have to buy nearly *all* new clothing, or alter what you have after any procedure that affects your body shape or weight.

- Be aware you will lose money if you cancel.

"Some women buy jewelry. Others get a mink. Or you can get a face-lift. It depends on what you choose to spend your money on ."

LISA, A BEAUTICIAN

1998 Range of Physician/Surgeon Fees* Per Procedure

Procedure	REG 1–2	REG 3–4	REG 5	REG 6–7	REG 8–9	National Average
Abdominoplasty (tummy tuck)	$4,627	$3,568	$4,086	$3,935	$4,028	$4,058
Blepharoplasty (cosmetic eyelid surgery)	$2,534	$1,985	$2,228	$2,008	$2,129	$2,187
Botox injection	$477	$393	$419	$460	$397	$424
Breast augmentation	$3,352	$2,598	$2,983	$2,844	$3,255	$3,001
Breast lift	$3,682	$2,948	$3,495	$3,232	$3,694	$3,439
Breast reduction (women)**	$5,189	$4,698	$5,060	$4,946	$4,746	$4,936
Buttock lift	$3,406	$3,700	$3,885	$3,530	$3,546	$3,648
Cellulite treatment (mechanical roller massage therapy)	$294	$193	$646	$759	$836	$588
Cheek implants	$2,311	$1,812	$2,131	$1,816	$2,191	$2,085
Chemical peel	$907	$705	$768	$893	$842	$821
Chin augmentation	$1,620	$1,422	$1,457	$1,353	$1,519	$1,482
Collagen injection	$366	$402	$340	$326	$327	$347
Dermabrasion	$1,294	$1,255	$1,250	$1,092	$1,275	$1,243
Face-lift	$5,864	$4,298	$4,818	$4,580	$4,850	$4,895
Fat injection	$950	$821	$807	$1,008	$838	$872
Forehead lift	$3,117	$2,212	$2,350	$2,246	$2,646	$2,504
Gynecomastia, treatment of	$3,050	$2,276	$2,491	$2,458	$2,389	$2,534
Hair transplantation	$2,846	$3,414	$2,646	$3,675	$3,369	$3,123
Laser hair removal	$488	$450	$454	$325	$474	$452
Laser skin resurfacing	$2,623	$1,808	$2,152	$1,986	$2,630	$2,276
Laser treatment of leg veins	$582	$335	$378	$294	$364	$406
Lip augmentation (other than injectable materials)	$1,281	$964	$1,353	$1,346	$1,493	$1,353
Lipoplasty (liposuction) (suction-assisted)	$2,521	$2,047	$2,226	$2,220	$2,312	$2,266
Lipoplasty (liposuction) (ultrasound-assisted)	$2,793	$2,340	$2,665	$2,100	$2,799	$2,562
Lower body lift	$5,431	$5,359	$4,773	$6,978	$4,790	$5,377
Otoplasty (cosmetic ear surgery)	$2,778	$2,052	$2,379	$2,327	$2,351	$2,374
Rhinoplasty (nose reshaping)	$3,791	$2,797	$3,389	$3,148	$3,296	$3,304
Sclerotherapy	$300	$237	$295	$224	$267	$269
Thigh lift	$4,020	$3,533	$3,479	$3,460	$3,239	$3,516
Upper arm lift	$3,088	$2,557	$2,599	$2,658	$2,493	$2,643

*Figures are for physician/surgeon fees only and do not include fees for surgical facility, anesthesia, medical tests, prescriptions, surgical garments, or other miscellaneous costs realated to surgery. Figures for procedures often performed on more than one body site in the same session reflect typical fees for one site.

**Breast reduction may be covered by insurance, depending on the patient's breast size, body type, and symptoms. Fees may vary.

The regional breakdowns used in the above table are as follows:
REG 1—New England (CT, ME, MA, NH, RI, VT)   REG 4—West North Central (IA, KS, MN, MO, NE, ND, SD)   REG 7—West South Central (AR, LA, OK, TX)
REG 2—Middle Atlantic (NJ, NY, PA)   REG 5—South Atlantic (DE, DC, FL, GA, MD, NC, SC, VA, WV)   REG 8—Mountain (AZ, CO, ID, MT, NV, NM, UT, WY)
REG 3—East North Central (IL, IN, MI, OH, WI)   REG 6—East South Central (AL, KY, MS, TN)   REG 9—Pacific (AK, CA, HI, OR, WA)

We are talking about a serious chunk of change here. By far, the vast majority of women choosing surgery *aren't* rich. They work for a living, and work hard. They're retailers and teachers, hair stylists and manicurists, nurses (*lots* of nurses!) and social workers. So how do they come up with the money to pay for their surgeries?

First of all, girlfriend, you *can* afford cosmetic surgery . . . if, as girlfriend Lisa said, it's what you choose to save, work overtime, borrow, or blackmail to get. *Blackmail?* Not exactly—the real situation is pressing a husband's guilt button, but more on that later. So what follows are some of our girlfriends' deepest secrets—the clever, devious, and downright sneaky ways they covered costs.

Visa, Mastercard, American Express . . . or all of the above.

The girlfriend pulled out her wallet and handed over several credit cards. "Let's see . . . put $500 on this one; $1,500 on my Visa gold; another $2,000 on my Discover card. And I'll write a check for $300." It's not fiction. Many women use up to five cards, putting part of the cost on each one. Don't be embarrassed, your surgeon's office is used to it. We guarantee you won't be the first to do it.

Or have you gotten a new major credit-card offer in the mail? Many girlfriends have considered the invitation for a "pre-approved" card as a sign that the time is now to get the surgery they've been dreaming of. Frankly, if you can get an annual percentage rate of 3.9, 5.9, or 9.9 percent, it may be the most economical way to go—cheaper than a bank loan, with less red tape.

Best bet for borrowing to pay: a very-low-interest credit card.

Loans.

Most cosmetic surgeons will help you finance surgery through a lending institution. (If you don't blink about paying for your husband's new pickup truck or a trendy Jeep Cherokee, what is so terrible about getting a bank loan to do something just for you?)

Don't be shy about asking if your surgeon has a loan plan available. Many of them do.

Don't overlook personal loans from family members—especially parents.

What about those special loan companies set up just to cover plastic surgery? You might see their ads in upscale magazines. Here's the real deal: Most surgeons will not work with these loan agencies because they require a high percentage, not only in interest from the patient, but they want an 8 or 9 percent payment of the total cost *from the doctor.* Either the doctor has to take less for the procedure than if you paid directly (highly unlikely), or charge you more to cover the added cost. Either way, most surgeons just say no.

Divorce settlements, insurance windfalls, and yes, death benefits.

Divorce is one of the biggest catalysts for a woman's decision to have surgery . . . and one of the ways to pay for it if you have a good lawyer. If your ex has dumped you for a twenty-six-year-old, or has been keeping a mistress in Peoria, it's only justice. Let him eat his heart out when he sees you looking drop-dead beautiful.

Speaking of dropping dead, the passing away of a husband also brings many women to surgery. Despite women's liberation and growing independence, burying a spouse often is what actually releases a wife to do what she's wanted to do for years. Free at last . . . and with his insurance policy to play with.

Then there are cheating husbands.

Girlfriend X, who ended up with a face-lift, blepharoplasty, Botox injections, abdominoplasty, rhinoplasty, laser, and liposuction, says, "I caught him. I hired a private detective, and I had the proof that he was having an affair. Then I got a damn good lawyer. I suppose, inside, I may never get over that feeling of betrayal. If you haven't experienced it, you cannot imagine how it feels when everything you believe in turns out to be a lie.

I made my husband move out—and I stayed in our house with our children. No matter how miserable and lonely I felt inside, no matter how much I wanted him and our marriage back, I didn't bend. I gave him terms.

If he wanted back into our marriage, he had to agree to marital counseling, a complete severing of all ties to the bitch—no exceptions—and all the money I needed for cosmetic surgery.

My advice? Girlfriends, you have a backbone and a brain. Use them both.

Raising money with special projects.

Don't overlook your entrepreneurial instincts. Take on part-time work specifically to raise the money you need—or start a small business on the side.

Hold garage sales or sell items at a flea market. (You can also sell things for friends who don't have the time or space. Be straightforward about the fact you need to take a commission of 15 to 25 percent to pay for your time and effort. Most girlfriends will be thrilled that they have a "retail" outlet for their extra stuff.)

Take the expensive wedding gift you keep in the closet to an auction (the auction house will take a commission, but this is "found" money), or sell it through a newspaper ad.

Sell your collectibles or vintage clothing at an on-line auction. Only do this *if* you have a scanner or digital camera and a personal Web site (your on-line server usually provides one free); otherwise forget it. The biggest and best on-line auction is www.ebay.com.

What won't work.

Don't try bartering—you know: "I'll clean your house for the next five years in exchange for a face-lift."

Don't try negotiating with the doctor. You will lose your pride and you won't get anywhere.

"In my family, it is acceptable to spend money on furniture, a big house, a luxury car, or a trip to Disneyworld. But cosmetic surgery—it's unthinkable! Isn't feeling good about myself more important than putting new wall-to-wall carpeting down in the living room?"

GLORIA, HOSPITAL NURSE

But what about insurance?

Girlfriends, here comes that old saying, "There's some good news and there's some bad news."

The good news is many insurance companies will pay for all or part of two expensive procedures, abdominoplasty or breast reduction, *if* they are causing a medical problem. You need to ask your doctor about this.

An insurance company might pay for an upper blepharoplasty if your vision is being hampered by the excess skin. However, you must take a test to prove this; and it is most often approved for older women in their sixties and seventies. Some younger girlfriends do meet the test, so it's worth looking into if you have a serious "droop." Any eye surgery strictly for cosmetic reasons will *never* be covered.

What about nose jobs? If your nose has been injured (*not* years ago!), the repairs will be covered. If you have a breathing problem because of a deviated septum or other defect, all or part of the surgery may be covered. However, any part of the surgery performed for aesthetic reasons will *not* be covered.

The removal of moles and cysts are usually covered, including their biopsies.

The bad news is, girlfriends, for any surgery to enhance or change your looks, you are the primary, and only, payer.

The Best Advice

Denise Zawilla said to tell all girlfriends: "Don't ever kick yourself in the ass over the money you spent on plastic surgery."

We agree. When you feel better about yourself, your whole life is affected in a positive way. The "ripple effect" is a tidal wave through every aspect of your life—including how you treat those you love—and, most of all, how you treat yourself.

Money can't buy happiness . . . but it can buy cosmetic surgery.

PREPARING FOR SURGERY AND RECOVERING AFTERWARD

Time is on your side when it comes to plastic surgery. No one's rushing you. You need time to get your body ready, to put your mind in the right place, to dramatically cut your risks, and to take the stress out of recuperating. You need to plan. You need to take control. You need *two months* to get ready for any of the big surgeries! More time won't hurt; less might be okay for breast augmentation, the facial implants, blepharoplasty, brow-lifts, or modest amounts of liposuction. Most surgeries, however, are planned long in advance because of your doctor's busy schedule. However, if the doctor has a cancellation and you get a call to see if you want to move up the date, think twice. Don't rush into the operating room. Your body doesn't detoxify, heal, firm up, or slim down quickly. The only thing a girlfriend's body does overnight is gain weight.

PREPARING YOUR BODY

Your doctor may give you specific things to do for your procedure. Tape them on the refrigerator and follow them to the letter. Here is our general advice:

- To diet or not to diet. You should maintain your current weight—unless you are having a face-lift. If you are having a lift, lose as much weight as possible before surgery. Your face sags most after weight loss.

- Stop smoking. At the minimum, you have to stop smoking for two weeks before surgery and for two weeks afterward. If possible, kick the habit earlier, so you are not stressed by trying to get off nicotine as well as recovering from the surgery. If you have tried to quit before and failed, get some nicotine gum or the inhaler to help you out when you are about to reach for a cigarette. These over-the-counter aids might get you through the rough spots. We researched the nicotine patch, and you *cannot* use it before or after surgery. The high, steady dose of nicotine can be harmful and impede your recovery.

  Smokers, you have to face facts. Some doctors won't operate on you if you are smoking. *Don't lie!* Susan has seen girlfriends taking a last puff right before they came through the facility's door. *By lying about smoking, you are exposing yourself to the risk of disfigurement and death.* We can't pretty up that truth for you.

  Here is the nitty-gritty: Smoking makes your skin die. If you have a face-lift, smoking can kill the skin on your face over a large area. It can keep incisions from healing. It will make your scarring worse.

  Smoking can kill you by causing a blood clot. Both nicotine and carbon monoxide will increase the stickiness of your blood.

  Smoking will slow your recovery and increase your suffering by contributing to edema (swelling).

- Stop drinking alcohol at least two weeks before and two weeks after your surgery. If you tend to drink regularly, detoxify yourself over a longer period. If you need some help from your doctor on this, get it.

The same advice applies to any dependence on, or recreational use of, drugs.

- Avoid the following vitamins, herbs, and foods for a minimum of two weeks before and after surgery. Check the labels of all medications, including cough syrups. We recommend you stay away from these blood-thinning substances for even longer, especially vitamin E.

Drugs, Herbs, and Foods to Avoid Before and After Surgery

- Anticoagulants. Please check with your doctor before stopping.

- Antihistamines in cold and allergy pills.

- Aspirin. Even one aspirin tablet can impair platelet function for a month. If you accidentally take aspirin or an aspirin product, tell your doctor. Surgery may be postponed. Over-the-counter medications should be avoided. Prescription drugs can also contain aspirin.

- Foods that impede clotting including MSG-containing curried, Japanese, or Chinese foods, garlic, onions, soy products (including tofu), ginger, red pepper, purslane, muskmelon or cantaloupe, black tree fungus or Chinese mushrooms, wakame seaweed.

- Guaifenesin in certain cold medicines and cough syrups can lead to bleeding during and after surgery.

- Herbs and herbal teas that impede clotting including evening primrose, willow (salix), bilberry, sichuan lovage.

VITAMIN E (TOCOPHEROL) WARNING

Vitamin E is a potent blood thinner. You must stop all vitamin E intake as far in advance of your surgery as possible. Stop taking it even if you are just contemplating surgery. Protein shakes are often supplemented with vitamin E and diet drinks are laced with it, too. Watch out for vitamin E in

- energy and nutrition bars and meal-substitute shakes;

- soy products including drinks, tofu, and meat substitutes;

- processed foods, breakfast cereal, and bread;

- soaps, shampoo, and hand and body lotion;

- multivitamins and other supplements that include vitamin E.

Ask for a "bleed test" before your surgery if you have been taking supplements for many years.

PRE-SURGERY TIPS

■ Eat a balanced diet, with adequate calcium, protein, and iron. Green tea also strengthens capillaries and acts as an antioxidant.

■ Start walking. As little as thirty minutes three times a week will improve your circulation and help improve your health.

- Hormones should be stopped one week before surgery. Please check with your doctor before stopping. You do not need to stop taking birth-control pills.

- Ibuprofen.

- Nutritional supplements including vitamin E, any multivitamin or antioxidant formula, fish oil capsules, Omega-3 capsules, garlic capsules, evening primrose oil, GLA (gamma-linolenic acid).

You Can Take . . .

- Some painkillers—so check with your doctor, all antibiotics, all vitamins except vitamin E, high-blood-pressure pills, heart pills, iron tablets, ulcer pills, antacids, thyroid pills, contraceptives, some muscle relaxants, eye medications, and acetaminophen (Tylenol or Tylenol ES).

- 500 mg of vitamin C, with bioflavoids if possible, twice a day for two weeks before surgery. Some doctors also recommend arnica montana homeopathic remedy and vitamin K (this needs a prescription) beginning the week before surgery.

Prepare Yourself Mentally

Your mind has a powerful effect on your recovery. Your attitude has a measurable impact on how well your surgery turns out. To build up your mental health, we recommend the following activities and exercises.

- Research your procedure thoroughly.

- Once you schedule your surgery, stay away from "toxic" people who are negative about your surgery. Instead, develop a support system of positive people you feel comfortable talking to about your plans.

- If you are feeling any anxiety, get relaxation tapes or affirmation tapes, and begin regular breathing exercises. If you have concerns or questions about your surgery, make sure you get answers.

- Have reasonable expectations. Be clear about the results you can expect from your surgery. Reinforce the idea that you must be patient. You will not see the results you want until you heal and the swelling subsides . . . and it can take months.

- Promote a relaxed atmosphere in your life. Deal with environmental stress. As the day for your surgery approaches, try to arrange your schedule so that anything you find extremely stressful is eliminated. For instance, don't schedule a dentist appointment the week before surgery. Don't plan to see your accountant. Don't have guests. Screen your phone calls. Plan to go into surgery well-rested.

- Realize there *is* a mind-body connection. Your attitude *does* influence the outcome of surgery. Patients who go into surgery feeling confident, positive, and eager have a faster recovery and fewer complications.

- Get a book of affirmations. Say them to yourself daily. Create your own as well, including: "I feel strong and healthy"; "I feel confidence in my surgeon"; "My surgery is going to go well—and I am going to look terrific"; "I am going to care about myself first—and only then can I truly care about others without resentment and anger"; "My happiness is important"; "Feeling good about the way I look is important"; "I will reach my goals"; "My dreams are important"; and "My health comes first!"

Prepare for Your Recovery

Too many women we know don't get their affairs in order before going into surgery. Girlfriends, surgery takes as much, or more, planning than the biggest party you have ever thrown or the longest vacation. You can't wait until the week—or the day—before your operation to start getting ready. Your recovery will go more smoothly, you will have fewer complications, *and your results will be better* if you carefully plan the days before and after your surgery. Here are some of the tips our girlfriends recommend:

- Arrange for adequate time away from your job. *Have a contingency plan ready in case you cannot go back as soon as you anticipate because of a complication.*

- If you have a family to care for, arrange for babysitters and caregivers.

    If you are having a tummy tuck, face-lift, or other "serious" surgery, try to arrange for children to stay elsewhere for the first three to four days, at minimum. Why? They may be upset by your appearance; they can accidentally cause you injury; and you need to focus on yourself and your recovery, not on caring for someone else. Children are by nature "needy." You cannot fulfill their needs after your surgery. Get someone else to do the job.

- Put together a "team" to handle your normal daily responsibilities. *List* them! This includes work *and* home. Please, don't put all your tasks and routines on your significant other. It's not fair—and it won't work. You don't need a resentful or exhausted partner when you are flat on your back and helpless.

- Arrange to have an overnight caregiver during the first forty-eight hours after surgery if you are not staying in a supervised facility.

After that, arrange for help while you convalesce at home. Your procedure will dictate the amount of assistance you need, but with most surgeries you *cannot* do housework for a week. (Ah, shucks.)

- Arrange for someone to drive you to and from your surgery, and for follow-up appointments until you are able to drive yourself. Or take a cab!

- Make sure you have completed all pre-surgery testing and/or have gotten your medical records to your surgeon.

- Fill all prescriptions for medications you will need after surgery.

- Buy small Dixie cups. Use them for each dose of your medication. Lay them out before you go in for surgery, labeled with the time and the day and containing the pills you need. This will help your caregiver—and you, since your brain will be foggy from the anesthesia.

- Buy bags of frozen peas (or refreezable ice packs), to use on swollen areas.

- Plan out what you will eat and drink the first forty-eight hours after surgery. Be sure you have plenty of fluids at hand.

- Get a humidifier if you are having a rhinoplasty.

ROID RAGE

If you are prescribed steroids, be aware that they make some people short-tempered, irritable, emotional, nervous, or high-strung. It is important for you to alert your caregiver to the possibility that you may not be your usual smiling, sunny self. Gloria became, in her words, "a raving lunatic," and drove everyone crazy with complaints, crying, and bouts of temper. You don't want a caregiver taking your behavior personally. You don't want to have a major battle with a spouse or lover. Warn them! If they see extreme "off-the-wall" emotional behavior on your part, they should alert your doctor to adjust your dosage or take you off the medication.

- Figure out what you are going to wear during your recovery. You may not have clothes that fit.

- Rent or buy videotapes to watch during your recovery (but no horror movies or thrillers that might raise your blood pressure!). Get fashion magazines to look at. If you like books, you might try books on tape. Best of all, get creative visualization tapes and use the power of your mind to speed your healing.

- Prepare your "recovery area." Set up your bed with the needed pillows or have your recliner ready with a little table beside it. Figure out how you will take care of normal bodily functions. Have everything ready before you come home from surgery.

- If you live alone, realize you will need help for the first forty-eight hours. Hire someone if you need to. Keep a cell phone handy.

- Face reality. If you cannot get rest or if you are going to have a relationship problem at home, arrange to stay elsewhere. You are going to be fragile and vulnerable. Treat yourself with care.

- Have a checklist for what you need to do the morning of your surgery. You will not be thinking clearly by then! Realize that you will be nervous, anxious, and wired. Write everything down.

A Note for Your Surgeon

If you have made an unusual or special request of your surgeon (you want a mole removed at the same time as your breast augmentation; you want your belly button a specific size; you want your areolae to remain large and not made smaller during your breast reduction)—*remind* your surgeon when you go in for the surgery. Yes, it is written on your chart, but if it is something extra or out of the ordinary—and realize it's probably been awhile since your consultation—don't be shy. *Speak out:* "Do you remember, we discussed removing the mole on my shoulder?" Or, since you may be groggy from a pre-op sedative, *write a note.* You are an equal partner. Don't expect your surgeon to remember what is of paramount importance to you. You will have to make your wishes known . . . more than once.

But I'm worried about the anesthesia!

Okay, you can handle getting ready for surgery—except for your fear of anesthesia. Many women have a terror of anesthesia. The best thing you can do is talk about your feelings with your doctor

WHAT TO WEAR TO SURGERY

Here's what to do and what not to do, to dress for the big day.

- *Do not* wear any article of clothing that has to go over your head.

- Don't wear a dress—unless it completely opens up in the front and is very loose, like a denim sundress.

- Don't wear pantyhose.

- Don't wear dress shoes. Since you may not be permitted to bend over and you might be a little dizzy, wear slip-on shoes, or have someone else lace up your sneakers (or wear them without laces). Forget socks if it's warm out.

- Whatever you do, *don't wear jeans!* The nurses hate them because they have to dress you after the operation, and it is nearly impossible to get jeans on an unconscious body. Remember, girlfriends, for most of us, jeans are a struggle to get on a *conscious* body.

- If you are small-breasted and don't have to wear a bra when you go out of the house, don't wear one to the operation.

- What you should wear: Best bet—a warm-up suit with loose, elastic-waist pants and a top that is *very loose*, washable, soft, and zips or buttons up the front. If the weather isn't too cold, the jacket to a warm-up suit will work beautifully. A dark color is a good idea in case there is seepage of blood and fluid from your incision(s).

and the nurses. But knowledge helps a great deal, too. Here is some essential information to ease your fears:

- Most cosmetic-surgery procedures are done under local anesthetic and intravenous sedation. If this is what you will be having, realize it's a "twilight sleep." You will be breathing on your own. You may be awake enough to be talking during the procedure, though you will not remember because you are given a drug that causes you to forget. The drugs are very short-lived, and wear off quickly (each dose only lasts about ten minutes, so you are given just a small amount over and over until the operation is over). And the drugs used now are very safe.

  Besides this "twilight sleep," other types of anesthesia used are spinal/epidural field blocks—which are very safe—and general endotracheal anesthesia. Inquire about what type you will have and why.

- Also, you will probably talk to the anesthesiologist shortly before your surgery. He or she can answer your questions and listen to your concerns; but keep in mind, lying on the table about to go under may not be the best time for a heart-to-heart conversation. Don't hesitate to ask to speak to the anesthesiologist in advance if you have deep-seated fears.

VITAMIN K TOPICAL CREAM

Yes, there is a way to make the bruises vanish more quickly after surgery (or anytime, especially if you bruise easily!). Many surgeons prescribe oral vitamin K before surgery to help your blood clot better. Afterward, vitamin K can help you, too, by rubbing it on the bruised area. Girlfriends who have used vitamin K cream after liposuction or facial surgery all say it helped them get rid of bruises, frequently within a week. When you are walking around in sunglasses to cover your two "black eyes," vitamin K cream can be a godsend! Ask your doctor about it before your surgery.

- Aftereffects of anesthesia vary widely from patient to patient. You might be wide-awake and cheery, hungry, and alert. You may be babbling on and on, a real Chatty Kathy. More likely you will be thirsty, groggy, and prone to lapses of memory for the first forty-eight hours. This is why it is a good idea to put your medication in little cups ahead of time! (Some girlfriends warned that the anesthesia "wiped them out" for an entire week.)

- Remember that nausea after surgery can now be controlled through the use of a suppository. You can ask about this ahead of time. If you do get nauseated, call your doctor.

Girlfriends, listen: "Death on the table" is extremely rare in cosmetic surgery. Every surgery carries a risk, but if you have put yourself in good hands and your health has been carefully evaluated, you will not go to sleep and *not* wake up. If you make sure your anesthesiologist is qualified and board-certified, you can put your worries to rest.

But, girlfriends, take charge! *You are responsible for your care.* Don't just go with the flow—direct the current.

GENERAL POST-OPERATIVE ADVICE

Most surgeons will give you a list of do's and don'ts for your safe recovery from a cosmetic-surgery procedure. But hear us on this one, girlfriends, there is no one set of rules. Some rules for recovery are generally agreed upon, others are controversial, and still others are changing month by month. *If you spot something in this book that your doctor didn't advise, ask about it before you try it.*

Most girlfriends we know who had problems after surgery caused them by doing something out of ignorance or arrogance. *Empower yourself with education, and never think you are an exception to the rule!*

For All Surgeries

In advance.

- Arrange for peace and quiet for two days after your surgery.

- Discourage visitors.

- Plan to watch television only if it will relax you. Watch no movies that will result in a release of adrenaline or increase your blood pressure. You may not be able to hold up a book to read comfortably, and you might have to rig something up. You might wish to get some books on tape instead.

- For all surgeries, you must have complete bedrest for forty-eight hours. (Usually, you may get up to go to the bathroom or even sit at the table to eat.)

After surgery.

- Food and drink: On the night after surgery, you can have sips of water, ice chips, or 7-Up or ginger ale. You may have decaffeinated Coke, juices, soup, and Jell-O, but avoid caffeinated tea and coffee. Eat a soft diet for supper if you feel up to it, but avoid greasy foods. *You do not want to get nauseous and vomit!* Coughing and vomiting can cause a hematoma (a collection of blood under the skin). Avoid alcohol for two weeks (before and after surgery).

THE BEST ICE PACK

We recommend you use frozen peas instead of ice packs. Get the peas in a flexible plastic pouch (not a box!). You can wrap the pouch in a dishtowel or place it in a man's sock. The temperature of the frozen peas will be perfect, it will contour to your face, and peas are inexpensive. Get several bags and refreeze as necessary. Corn will work, too, but because peas are round, they seem to be ideal. Real ice is too messy. Chemical ice packs may be too cold, too hard, and too expensive. Frozen peas are just right.

- Medication: *Follow your doctor's instructions to the letter.*

- You may also take 500 mg of vitamin C twice a day for two to four weeks. (You can take even higher doses if you can tolerate it. A sign of too high a dose is diarrhea.) Vitamin C with bioflavinoids is preferred. You can take *arnica montana* capsules for three days following surgery. These are available in the health-food stores. Vitamin K cream on bruises will speed healing.

- Apply ice packs. Ice greatly reduces swelling. Follow your doctor's instructions diligently. You can buy ice packs ahead of time at the drugstore.

  Remember—never put ice directly on your skin. You can actually injure yourself. You may be numb. Take extra care. Also, do not put any warm compresses on yourself until you test the temperature on the inside of your wrist. You can burn yourself.

Sleep tips.

- For almost all procedures, sleep on your back only.

- To help reduce the swelling after liposuction, sleep with your legs raised *above your heart level* for the first three to four weeks after surgery. Two or three pillows under your legs are helpful. (See Teresa's suggestion in chapter 4 for a great alternative to this.) Ace bandages wrapped from the base of the toes to the calves may also be helpful.

- After breast surgery or facial surgeries, sleep on two, three, or four pillows with your head elevated at all times. You may also sleep in a recliner with your head up. A pillow under each arm may make you more comfortable

- After a rhinoplasty, a cool-air humidifier in your bedroom will help keep your mouth moist and allow for a more restful sleep. Keep a glass of water by the bed. For the *first forty-eight hours* after surgery, sleep on two, three, or four pillows to minimize edema as much as possible. Keep your head elevated at all times. You might prefer to sleep in a recliner. Do not sleep with your head bent down toward your chest.

Personal hygiene.

- Have someone with you when you take your first shower! If you have been wearing "the garment," remember, it is a compression garment (like the pump-up trousers the EMTs carry for trauma victims). When you take it off for the first time, your blood pressure will drop as your blood rushes feetward. You will feel faint. Coupled with the warm water of the shower, you could go down with a bang. Put a chair in the shower, and have a girlfriend—or your sweetie—there to lean on.

Don'ts

- Do not take aspirin, Advil, Motrin, or vitamin E (see the complete list on pages 247–48).
- Do not smoke for two weeks after surgery.
- Do not lift objects (even if they are only moderately heavy).
- Do not push anything (i.e., do not run the vacuum cleaner or move furniture).
- Do not do general housework.
- Do not do anything that will raise your blood pressure: physical exertion, exercise, stress, or *sex!*
- Do not go back to the gym or engage in vigorous exercise until your doctor gives you the okay—no sooner than two weeks, and preferably after three weeks.
- Do not sunbathe until all bruising is gone.

- Don't rush your recovery. Don't get up on a chair and start hanging curtains or painting the bedroom ceiling.

Okay, girlfriends, now you know how to keep safe and how to speed your recovery. But do you know what you have to remember above everything? *Slow down.* You will feel terrific—but your body is healing. For two weeks you must not exert yourself, no matter how good you feel. Don't go on an all-day shopping binge. Don't start redecorating. Don't start cleaning out closets or doing load after load of wash. Don't stand in the kitchen making lasagne. Don't plant a garden. Don't get nervous about weight gain and start walking five miles. Sleep until you can't sleep another wink. Keep your feet up. Meditate. Watch the grass grow. *Take it easy for two full weeks. No exceptions. No one is allowed to cheat.* Now, link pinkies with us and promise.

SECRETS, LIES, OR FULL DISCLOSURE

Now we come to a major concern of many girlfriends, the one that makes even the terror of dying under anesthesia look like a hangnail: how to keep people from finding out you had cosmetic surgery.

Susan and Charlee both opt for full disclosure—most of the time. Every girlfriend who has taken this route found support everywhere for her decision, and was besieged by questions from other women who were thinking about it themselves. Outside of their own family, they encountered little or no disapproval. Barbara S. said the ladies in her altar society at church loved her upper blepharoplasty (eyelid surgery)—and this is a very conservative group of Polish Catholics. Sheri had the supermarket checkers following her weight-loss procedures with the intensity provoked by the latest tabloid story—or a Richard Simmons infomercial. They loved it!

But no one tells all of the people all of the time. There are people who just don't need to know. If you want *no one* to know, it's your call. You don't owe anybody an explanation. So we're going to tell you how our girlfriends coped with this dilemma—the strategies, the attitudes, the lies.

First of all, decide ahead of time whom you will tell and what you are going to say if confronted by your worst high-school enemy in the supermarket line, who says, "Well, you're looking good. What did you do, have a face-lift?"

You say, "Well, thank you! I'm on a strict diet and vitamin plan that I got from my nutritionist. No red meat. No sugar. Guess it's working. She's out on the West Coast, but let me know if you want her name; you look a little tired."

Get the idea? Create your cover story (we'll give you some below), and don't be taken unawares. Remember, you can say outrageous things to perfect strangers who say something to you. Be wild, be creative. It's none of their business to start with!

Besides strangers, people you know will ask about your changed appearance. You need to be ready to answer them, with great conviction.

But first, who should you tell?

TELLING YOUR CHILDREN

Girlfriends, first of all, don't expect your children to be supportive. If they are, terrific. Chances are, they won't be. Children don't want to see *any* change in you. They've been known to start bawling if you come home wearing a new pair of eyeglasses. Imagine how they'll react if you come home with a new nose. After her rhinoplasty, Cindy's two-year-old started screaming and refused to come near her for hours; the rejection hurt worse than her procedure.

So, dear girlfriends, let us now be totally frank with you about your children and your decision to have cosmetic surgery. First of all, this is a decision that is yours, not theirs. You are not going to lose their love if you look different. Do not—we repeat, *do not*—solicit your children's opinions about whether to have surgery or not. Not only are you *not* going to get the answer you want to hear, it puts them in an inappropriate role. You are the parent. Children do not have the capacity to handle adult decisions. Younger children, even teenagers, have no understanding of the reasons you are contemplating a procedure. They have little life experience. Besides, by nature, children are egocentric. That means, because they are children, their thoughts focus on themselves: "What is going to happen to *me* if my mom dies . . . if she can't take care of me . . . if she is so pretty someone will fall in love with her and take her away from me?" They are not going to think about what is best for Mom. Don't expect them to, and you won't be disappointed. And be prepared for some acting-out behavior, from all-out threats ("If you do that, I'm getting a tattoo") to tears.

If you have a loving, open friendship with your older children, you might find them right there with you, cheering you on when you have a face-lift. But don't bet on it. Mother-daughter relationships, especially, are deep, complex, and often explosive. Liz told one daughter, but another—who lives twenty minutes away from her—never knew about Liz's face-lift, liposuction, or mini-lift six years after the first procedure. Her daughter never even noticed. Impossible? Children, dear girlfriends—even loving, grown children—can be incredibly self-centered when it comes to you, their giver of unconditional love.

Here is the verdict from most girlfriends: If you have to give any explanation at all, tell your children you are having a procedure done for a medical reason. If you are having a nose job, you need correction of a breathing problem; a tummy tuck is a "woman's problem"; liposuction is a circulation problem—or whatever your imagination dreams up. (Breast augmentation may present a challenge!) Don't feel guilty. Don't feel hypocritical: "But I always told my children lying is the worst thing you can do!" That philosophy works fine for a grade-schooler, but real life is not so black-and-white.

And for heaven's sake, don't let the children see you when you are swathed in bandages in the first days after a lift. They will be scared to death. Spare them the trauma of seeing you "out of it" after a tummy tuck. Send them to Grandma's. Send them anywhere. But don't have them on the premises.

TELLING YOUR RELATIVES

Girlfriend Teresa says, "Don't—especially if they're Italian." Well, it doesn't really matter if they are Italian, Jewish, Polish, or Irish. You know where their values lie. Teresa explained that in her family, who emigrated to America from Sicily after World War Two, spending money on material things, including the plastic-covered living-room furniture, was acceptable; spending thousands on cosmetic surgery would get you an eyeroll to heaven and a torrent of hysterical Italian tirades from every widowed aunt in black.

You owe no relative—except perhaps a parent—any explanation at all.

You don't need the phone gossip line to start buzzing with you as the subject. But that can happen, so get your head together and don't let it bother you. Get your own version circulating (recruit a ringer, like your closest cousin, to start the story). Here's an example: "A face-lift? No, that's not what happened. Poor Linda! She had this terrible cyst on her cheek. Totally benign, but what an operation! *Mama mia.* She's so lucky the doctor did such a terrific job!"

Now, here's a word about telling your parents. Girlfriends, nearly 100 percent of the women we talked to said the disapproval they expected from their parents never happened. There was lots of concern, but parents offered total support in the end. In fact, many parents became the biggest cheerleaders.

You see, dear girlfriends, once your parents know that you are okay physically after the surgery, they also see that you are happy. If you had been down in the dumps about yourself before your procedure, you are now radiant and thrilled. When a mom sees her child happy, that's what matters to her. Initially it may be hard to tell them (and you might want to wait until after the surgery is over), but if they always stood behind you before, they will be there now.

Here are the stats on the reactions of other family members: Biggest criticisms came from cousins, aunts, and *any in-laws*. Sisters usually decide they want to do what you did, especially younger sisters. Brothers never notice.

Telling Friends and Coworkers

The most virulent opposition and the greatest jealousy you will encounter may be from "friends." Before the surgery they will try to talk you out of it. Afterward, they may scrutinize your results and criticize the job the surgeon did. Many years ago, after Susan had a blepharoplasty, one so-called friend looked at her and remarked: "You know, one of your eyebrows is higher than the other." The procedure didn't change Susan's eyebrows in any way. One was higher than the other before surgery, but the "friend" didn't know that. The remark was pure catiness.

Some girlfriends tell one best friend. Some girlfriends tell none.

You are under no obligation to tell *anyone* but your significant other . . . and maybe even not him (at least not the *whole* truth).

Depending on where you work, your coworkers may never know. Or they may be gathering around you in the recovery room, dying for a peek.

Decide ahead of time who should know—and who shouldn't.

Be prepared—and we mean this—be prepared for jealousy from other women. Develop a thick skin. Remember that their remarks are coming from envy—and, very likely, hurt and bad feelings about themselves. If you are fifty and turning heads, getting whistles, and have maître d's rushing over to seat you, your friend—whose birthday is two months before yours and who has just been mistaken for your mother—is not going to feel very good about herself. You might opt for compassion and ask her if she'd like to know how to get surgery of her own.

Of course, that remark could press a button to set off emotional fireworks. But then, you might really enjoy the whole show! Susan remembers being "attacked" at a party by a friend. "I'd *never* get surgery," she insisted. "It's vain! It means you just can't accept yourself! It's feeding the false values of our culture!" The tirade went on and on. Six months later the girlfriend was in Susan's office for a consultation. Three surgeries later—and the girlfriend is now a traffic-stopping brunette—they laugh about *"never."*

TELLING YOUR SIGNIFICANT OTHER

Telling your husband, future husband, or lover is a complex issue. First, do you tell him the truth? Second, do you tell him how much your surgery really costs? A girlfriend, who requested her name be withheld, related, "I lied about how much the liposuction cost. Then when I went back for the second procedure, I told him the doctor had to fix something about the first one and it wasn't costing anything. He never knew I spent over $5,000."

Susan has, on numerous occasions, been asked by girlfriends to send an "official" letter about upcoming surgery for a vaguely alluded-to medical problem. The girlfriend then leaves the letter in a conspicuous place before telling her husband she has to get her female organs fixed (tummy tuck), needs sinus work (rhinoplasty), has a vision problem (blepharoplasty), and so on. One woman completely hid a butt tuck from her mate. We still haven't figured that one out.

Lots of women schedule liposuction when they know their husbands will be out of town for a few weeks. He just assumes she dieted, if he notices at all. (They often don't.)

Almost no woman tells her husband the actual cost of her surgery.

Many women have the full support and help of their husbands.

Many women, such as girlfriend X (see pages 242–43), have a guilt button to press.

But what about the future husband?

Dina had an interesting question. At what point in a relationship do you tell your boyfriend that you have breast implants? Are you obliged to reveal this before marriage? We asked a few men. They insisted they'd know anyway. (Yeah, right, fellows.) They thought they should be told only if there was the possibly it posed a future health problem. None of them cared whether a woman would be able to breast-feed a child or not after surgery. They didn't even want to think about breast-feeding (this may relate to a territorial instinct about those breasts being theirs, not some future child's meal ticket).

Our conclusion: Don't tell if you don't want to. He won't know.

Apart from breast implants, which may turn into a raging philosophical debate, you do not have to reveal any other surgery to a future mate or steady boyfriend. Do you feel it necessary to disclose that you had your wisdom teeth removed . . . or your gall bladder? Do you tell him, "Well, I first changed my hair color at sixteen"?

If you must confess, tell your shrink or your priest. If you want to tell your lover, accept the responsibility that it may be used against you in a future argument . . . or after you break up. This is a serious consideration. Unless you are going to marry the man, *do not tell him anything!*

Strategies and Cover Stories

- Many girlfriends suggested that you change your hair color or hairstyle at the same time as your face-lift (or any other procedure). People will notice something is different and immediately will assume it's your hair. You will hear, we promise, "That color looks *great* on you."

- Learn to say, "Thank you," graciously to the comment, "You look terrific," and don't explain anything!

- Dieting and weight loss explains your new contours from liposuction, a tummy tuck, or any other body surgery.

- Best cover stories for boobs: a side effect of medication; a result of hormone therapy; a result of weight gain; a family trait of late maturity; it happened after pregnancy.

- Best cover stories for facial bruises and swelling: a minor car accident, especially getting hit by the airbag; a home accident; or—the most common—dental work!

- Best cover stories for the rejuvenated look after a face-lift: a spa vacation; a nutritional program; acupressure therapy for migraines; weight loss; yoga classes; a new moisturizer.

- Cover stories for nose jobs: correction of a "breathing problem;" correction of a broken nose from an earlier injury; sinus trouble; a sports accident. No one ever just gets a nose job—trust us on this one: They all just had a deviated septum repaired.

Girlfriends, remember that whatever you say, people will believe it if you sound sincere; if you say it with conviction; if you don't go on and on with a long story; if you don't sound defensive—and if you are ready with your answer. People are terribly gullible. You can make up something totally outrageous, and people will believe you. Advertisers do it every day.

Last, dear girlfriends, you can't control what people think. You can't control what they say. You can only deal with how you feel. If you feel good about your surgery and your decision, even the meanest, cattiest remark will make you smile . . . because you will know it is pure envy speaking.

Through the Looking Glass: Life After Surgery

Susan has seen it over and over again. A woman comes in for a consultation. She sits in the chair on the opposite side of Susan's desk. Her clothes, often in neutral tones, often loose and layered, are chosen to avoid calling attention to her body. Her shoulders are hunched forward, her eyes are down, her fingers are busy picking at her skirt, her voice is low, shaky, and sad. Her body language announces, *I don't feel very good about myself.*

The same woman returns after surgery. She strides down the hall like it's a fashion-show runway, her hair is carefully done, her makeup is impeccable. A huge smile beams hello to the nurses. Electricity charges the air around her. An aura of luscious perfume precedes her. Her voice is strong, upbeat; her eyes are bright. Everything about her says, *I feel great. I look great. Here I come, world!*

It doesn't take psychological analysis to recognize what is obvious. The major impact of having a cosmetic-surgery procedure is to boost a woman's self-esteem. It is like getting a large inheritance. You can put it in the bank and not overtly alter your lifestyle, but you have the security of knowing it's there. Or you can go out and flaunt it.

Improved self-esteem has a domino effect in a woman's life. She copes better. She makes changes. She takes risks. She treats those she loves better. Charlee also believes that being attractive, having confidence, and developing a sense of presence puts women in a position of power—in relationships and in the workplace—and research is now supporting that idea.

Of course, external change isn't enough. However, the physical improvements created by cosmetic surgery can act as a catalyst for internal change. Some women, like Raquel, who had been through one major kick in the head after another, do not completely internalize their transformation. Their self-image lags behind their actual appearance. Getting used to looking gorgeous may take a little time. But it is a whole lot easier to feel you are worthy when your phone starts ringing and the fellow you met while you were walking your dog that morning is asking you out for dinner...when your boss sends you to California to clinch a major deal...when your boyfriend shamelessly shows you off to his family...when total strangers compliment you on your appearance.

A number of girlfriends did leave their marriages, got over a lost lover with a new man, found new jobs, or went to the beach for the first time—in a bathing suit—in twenty years.

And for every girlfriend, there was one universal aftereffect of having had a cosmetic-surgery procedure. Every single girlfriend went back for more. "It's addicting!" said Lisa. "It's addicting!" said Barb.

Susan explains that how often we have procedures depends on our "vanity quotient." Some women can wait ten years before they do a second procedure. Others are on the yearly maintenance plan. And we all are tempted by new products and techniques. The "lunchtime peel"? "Girlfriend, you *have* to try it." Subdermal massage? If you have a Visa card with enough available credit, why not! Lower-lid surgery? What are you waiting for—to look like a basset-hound?

For some girlfriends, the change surgery brings is subtle. For others it is dramatic and life-changing. But for every girlfriend there is a change, outside and in. And for one unforgettable girlfriend, the change was everything . . .

THE JOURNEY OF MARIANNE KOREY

At five o'clock on a Friday night, too early for the weekend crowd, an hour when just a few men and women stop off for a beer on their way home from work, Charlee walked into the half-light of Joe's Grotto, the local sports bar in Harvey's Lake, Pennsylvania. She was meeting a woman she had spoken to on the phone the day before. The woman had a musical voice, a bit sultry, sophisticated, worldly. Charlee had no idea what she looked like. "I'm blonde and about five-four," Charlee had said as she ended the phone call. The woman had laughed and said, "Well, I'm blonde and five-seven. I guess we'll find each other. And I'll be wearing a green Hawaiian shirt."

Susan had said that this woman was someone Charlee *had* to interview, that Marianne Korey was a woman whose life had been transformed by radical new procedures in cosmetic surgery. Charlee was excited that Marianne had agreed to speak to her; that, in fact, she *wanted* to tell her story. But what that story was, Charlee had no idea. None at all.

Now, from the far side of the island-style bar, which could have been a duplicate of the one on *Cheers,* a blonde-haired woman waved at Charlee, got up from the bar, picked up her handbag and a fruit-filled drink, and gestured that they should sit at a nearby table. She was a striking-looking woman, athletic: Her body was muscular and toned, not model-thin. Her welcoming smile was wide in a face that was classically Polish, from its perfect triangular shape to the slight tilt to her ice-blue sparkling eyes.

"I'm Marianne," she said, and shook Charlee's hand. Her grip was firm. Nothing about her was tentative. She was a definite presence in the large, still-mostly-empty room. "I'm so flattered you want to talk to me. I want so much to do something for other women, women like me."

Women like Marianne? Charlee didn't know what she meant. As Charlee slid onto a chair and put her folder on the small table, she expressed her thanks for Marianne's time and willingness to share her experiences, and told Marianne about Susan's insistence that Marianne be interviewed.

"I think the world of Susan and Dr. Collini," Marianne said. "I would do anything I could for them. They are part of a miracle, you see." And with that Marianne opened her wallet and took out a small, worn picture, no more than three by two inches. She put it down on the table in front of Charlee.

It was the picture of a young woman Charlee didn't recognize—a woman whose deep-set eyes were set in a wide face—a woman whose body was large, so large that her waist had to be half as wide as her height.

Charlee felt bewildered. She looked up at Marianne, who was vividly pretty, youthful, her face unlined, her eyes dazzling. There was no resemblance between her and the person in the picture—not in the face, not in the body, not in the sadness emanating from the girl who stood uncomfortably looking into the camera like a doe caught in a car's headlights, wanting to flee but frozen with fear.

"That was me three years ago," she said. "I weighed 340 pounds in that picture. That was the summer before my accident," she said, her throat catching with emotion. And then she told her story.

White female. Thirty-one years old. Morbidly obese.

Those words topped Marianne's medical chart. She lay in a hospital bed with a shattered ankle, but "morbidly obese," not the badly fractured bone, was listed as her condition. "Morbidly obese" were the words that defined how she had been treated for most of her life; they defined her identity in the eyes of the medical profession and in the eyes of the world.

"Fatty, fatty."

The kids at school had chanted the words over and over. Even if she covered her ears, she could hear the words, and the laughter. It was 1974. Wilkes Barre's winters are damp and cold, but even in the chill, the wide playground of St. Stanislav's grammar school was swarming with children. Marianne stood alone among the clusters of running boys and girls, her bulk even bigger under her down jacket and snowpants, her hands stuffed into mittens, a hat her mother had knit tied under her plump chin. She could barely move. It wasn't hard to tip her over. One quick little shove, and down she went on her behind, the momentum tipping her backward until her head hit the asphalt and she stared up at the gray sky. The children gathered around, and she could see their faces above hers. She struggled to sit up. She couldn't. She rolled over onto her belly. She tried to get on her knees but as soon as she did, someone would push her from the side and she'd roll over on her back again. The kids laughed. "Marianne's a whale! Marianne's a walrus!" Then someone jumped on her. Then someone else. "Marianne's a trampoline! Marianne's a trampoline!" they yelled. Sometimes in dreams she still feels the weight of them jumping.

Gentle, sensitive, deeply religious, unable and unwilling to fight back, the cruel taunts hurt more than the pushing and the jumping. Marianne could not escape them. In fact, she could not even run. She had never played softball. Or kickball. Or volleyball. She couldn't ride a bicycle. She couldn't even walk far without losing her breath—and besides, the insides of her thighs rubbed together. It was uncomfortable.

Once she had been pushed into the janitor's closet at school while her classmates screamed they wouldn't let her out until she lost weight. They locked the door from the outside and left, laughing. It was dark. She was terrified. It was long after school ended for the day before the janitor came along and heard her crying.

Food was comfort. Food was love. Food filled the emptiness inside.

Books helped fill her mind. Marianne read voraciously. She wanted to go to college; her grades were so good she had graduated at age fifteen. She had a scholarship, but she couldn't face the emotional drain of continuing in the school system. Besides, her financial help would be welcome at home, and Marianne was a giver, a caretaker, a young woman who put the needs of others before her own.

Now, just sixteen when she got a full-time job, she was quick-witted, eager, a hard worker—and weighed over two hundred pounds. Marianne took advantage of her knowledge of computers and landed a terrific position. But hiding behind a computer screen didn't fulfill her need to be with people. She loved helping others; with her inexhaustible patience and her empathy, she was good at it.

Soon she became a systems analyst. She studied public speaking and gained confidence. Her company loved her work. Did her weight hurt her as a professional? "I had to work twice as hard as everyone else to prove myself—as a woman. Then, twice as hard again to prove myself—as an obese woman," she said.

Teasing from coworkers went on nonstop. Comments were cruel. It was almost as if no one thought she had the same feelings as everyone else. Once, while standing with a coworker, she heard her boss yell, "Hey, I need you over here." When she began walking in his direction, she was greeted with the loud comment, "I don't want the fat one; I want the thin one." Everyone in the office laughed.

Marianne thought of Shylock in *The Merchant of Venice:* " 'If you prick us, do we not bleed? If you tickle us, do we not laugh? If you poison us, do we not die? And if you wrong us, shall we not revenge?' " The only revenge Marianne took was on herself. She retreated inside her mind, to a place that she thought of as a black room. There, she was away from the world—sheltered, safe, and yet trapped by an interior darkness she couldn't escape.

One of the worst incidents over her weight concerned an important Canadian account for her company. Marianne had helped the Canadian business set up their computer system over the phone, but they had hit a difficult problem with their network and needed someone to fly up and be on-the-spot. Marianne was the logical person to go. She knew the client. She knew their needs. And she knew how to make their system work.

"You don't have the right *physical presence,*" her boss said, "I'm sending someone from sales and marketing."

The salesperson, a thin brunette, was dispatched to Canada. She was a pretty woman, but she couldn't help the business set up their computer network. The people in Canada wanted Marianne. They called Marianne's company and raised hell. "Where the hell is Marianne? We need someone who can do the goddamn job! Either get her up here by Monday, or we're going to a different vendor."

The humiliation began on the commuter flight. Marianne squeezed down the narrow aisle and into the seat. The armrests gouged into her side. The seatbelt sign went on. She helplessly held the two ends of the seatbelt, trying to figure out how to make them meet. They were at least a foot too short. The angular, thin-legged stewardess came down the aisle to make sure everyone had buckled up. She stopped at Marianne. Her lips pursed and her nose wrinkled as if she had a bad taste in her mouth. Without looking at Marianne's face or saying a word to her, the stewardess bellowed, so that everyone in the plane could hear, "We need the extension for this one!" Marianne's face flamed red with embarrassment.

Landing at the small municipal airport, Marianne pushed herself out of her seat, stood up, and grabbed her briefcase from the overhead compartment. Her bulk filled the aisle, and the passengers in the seats at the rear of the plane waited with impatience for her to finish. When she got to the door, she looked down the steep descent of the openwork metal staircase that had been pushed up to the plane. She gripped her briefcase hard with one hand, and grabbed the railing with white knuckles. Lumbering one step at a time downward, she was soon breathing hard and perspiring from the exertion. Her legs felt like dead logs after the flight. She was fighting the panic that she would fall. At the bottom of the flight, two blue-suited men waited. One held a sign saying, *Marianne.* She saw the questions on their astounded faces: *Is this fat person Marianne? Is this the woman with the kind, beautiful voice?* But the two suits quickly recovered their manners, and greeted her with typical Canadian graciousness.

The next upsetting moment occurred when the three of them arrived at the office building. At the center of a wide expanse of beige carpet, a beautiful spiral staircase soared gracefully upward, linking the two main floors of the company. For Marianne it was an insurmountable obstacle. She began to tremble. Her host took one look at the stairs, another at Marianne, and stopped midstride. "Er, um, Joe . . . why don't you go on ahead? Marianne and I will take the elevator." Marianne finished the sentence mentally: *because this fat person will never even fit between the railings and even if she did, she could never haul her weight up those stairs.* She felt humiliated and ashamed.

With her usual competence, professionalism, and sweet personality, Marianne soon solved their computer problems and won their respect. She visited their homes for dinner, they treated her like family, and they sent a huge bouquet of flowers back to her home office to surprise her on her return. But she remembered how their faces had looked in that first moment when they saw her. And each time she remembered, the pain came back to her heart.

"You have such a pretty face. . . ." were words she had heard all her life. And she also heard the unspoken words, *If only you weren't so fat.*

It wasn't as if she hadn't dieted. The Beverly Hills Diet; the Cabbage Diet; the Atkins Diet; macro-bionics; protein fasts; Slim-Fast; Diet Fuel; the Hawaiian Diet . . . Marianne tried them all. She'd lose fifty pounds and gain back sixty. In her early twenties, she once fasted her way to thinness—and was back up to three hundred pounds in months. After all that yo-yo dieting, especially the fast, her metabolism had slowed down to a crawl, and her thyroid had become underactive. Her family—her Mom's side is from Hungary and her Dad's folks come from Poland—favored the heavy, fat-filled food of the Old Country. By the time Marianne had turned thirty, permanent weight loss seemed impossible.

But Marianne tried. She wouldn't eat all day at work: no coffee breaks, no lunch. Not one morsel of food passed her lips. She was determined to prove that food didn't control her, that she didn't *have to eat*. When she got home in the evening, though, she was ravenous. Her body screamed for food. She'd eat halushki, pierogies, potato pancakes, ham, pork chops, burgers, and potato chips by the carload. She consumed at least 2,500 or 3,000 calories every night. The weight stayed on—and grew.

By the time she turned thirty, she had never had a boyfriend. She dreamed about dating, but felt awkward and shy around men. She loved to dance but she would rather die than venture out to a club. Fears of rejection and her weight ruled what she did and what she didn't do. She had friends and family; she traveled; she walked her dog every night. The years had slipped by. Marianne's life might have drifted along its lonely way, except for what happened on the night before Christmas Eve in 1995.

It was already after six, and the chain bookstore was crowded with Christmas shoppers. Marianne was exhausted. She had already made her purchases, but the girlfriend shopping with her wasn't quite finished. "I need to get you a card," Joellyn said, knowing that Marianne's birthday was just a few days away. "Since you're done, why don't you get the car? By the time you bring it around, I'll be checked out. It'll save some time. I'm beat."

"Yeah, me too. I'll be waiting outside in maybe five minutes." Marianne headed for the door as her girlfriend turned to the card display.

The air was frigid when Marianne stepped outside. The temperature was hovering in the teens and on the way down to the single digits. The wind blew her hair wildly and penetrated her jacket. All she could think about was getting to the car where she could turn on the heater.

Directly in front of the entrance to the bookstore, she stepped off the curb into the parking lot. She didn't notice the ice. Before she realized what was happening, her ankle turned, and she heard three distinct cracks. She fell backward. Pain more intense than anything she had ever experienced shot up her leg. She landed hard on her spine, but she barely felt that. She thought she was going to pass out from the pain in her ankle. She screamed, then began calling for help.

People ran out of the store. "What's happening out here?" someone asked.

"An old fat lady fell," a little boy said.

"Call 911," someone else yelled.

Marianne wasn't "old." She was going to be thirty-one on her coming birthday. But she weighed 340 pounds, a weight that obscured her pretty face with double and triple chins, broadened her features, robbed her of her youth. Now it was part of the reason she was badly hurt, and she knew it. White waves of blinding pain washed over her.

"Marianne! Get up!" her girlfriend said, having run out of the store to find Marianne lying on the asphalt.

"I can't get up," she said in a voice tight with pain. "It hurts. The bone is going to go through the skin if I move. I feel it."

She wanted to cry—oh, how she wanted to cry! But the tears were silent ones. She didn't want to make a scene. Most of all she didn't want to draw attention to herself so that people stared. Despite her effort, she moaned. She couldn't stop the sounds. They seemed to come from somewhere so deep inside, she couldn't find the source.

"Are you really hurt that bad?" her friend asked, worried now, but still deeply embarrassed by Marianne lying on the ground, her coat askew, her eyes pleading. "Are you sure you can't get up? I'll drive you to the doctor." Joellyn looked as if she'd rather be anywhere but here, shivering in the cold, feeling helpless and so uncomfortable at Marianne's being the focus of so much curiosity.

Marianne couldn't even answer. She saw the faces of people gathering around. No one spoke to her. No one asked to help. They simply stared at her. She felt like a freak.

A good twenty minutes later, the ambulance came screeching up. Two skinny young volunteer EMTs jumped out and ran over. When they saw her, they stopped dead. "What's the matter, lady?" one asked.

"My ankle. My ankle. I fell. It's broken. Bad. It hurts. Oh god, it hurts," she moaned.

"We can't lift that lady," one of them said to the other.

"No shit. She's got to be three hundred pounds. Better call in. See what they want us to do with this one."

They didn't touch her. They didn't even walk over to her. Marianne continued to lie freezing and shaking on the cold ground. The crowd just stared.

"She's too fat to get up anyway," somebody said, as if she couldn't hear them.

"Man, I never saw anybody that fat," another said.

"I did. I had an uncle like that. He died of diabetes. Young. Damn shame the way people let themselves go."

The two EMTs stood near the ambulance, waiting for some-one to call them back and tell them what to do. They smoked cig-arettes and ignored Marianne. Finally they climbed into the cab to get warm.

In agony, utterly humiliated, shivering uncontrollably, Mari-anne closed her eyes and began to pray. *Please God, let me die. I can't bear this. I don't want to live anymore. Nobody cares. I don't want to live. Take me, please take me.* Over and over, through the pain, she prayed, *Let me die, let me die.* She felt the blackness coming and she didn't care. At least the hurting would be over.

Suddenly a deep, kind voice said, "Miss, can you open your eyes? Look at me. Listen. It's going to be okay. I'm going to help you. Come on now, take a deep breath." A handsome, dark-haired man with kind blue eyes took her hand and felt for her pulse. Then he smoothed the hair back from her face and held her head for a moment, saying comforting words. Then he yelled to one of the EMTs, who had gotten out of the ambulance, "Hey, buddy, put some blankets on this woman, she's hypothermic!"

Marianne looked at the man crouching beside her. "Are you an angel?" she said, feeling light-headed and ready to pass out again.

"Nah, I'm just an off-duty fireman," he said with a smile. He looked directly into Marianne's eyes. "I heard about your plight on my truck radio. Don't worry, we'll get you to a hospital. It's going to be all right, I promise. You've been a very brave girl. Now, just hold on a few more minutes. It's going to be all right."

"Don't move me," she said frantically. "The bone is coming through my skin."

Experienced and calm, the fireman instructed the EMTs in immobilizing her leg. Then he helped them roll her onto a board and strap her to it. But they still couldn't lift her. The fireman called to the people standing around staring. "Hey, would some of you young guys over there help us with this? We need some help here."

"Hey man, I'm not breaking my back," a teenager laughed.

"Me neither," another man hooted.

No one moved. No one helped.

"Sons of bitches," Marianne heard the fireman mutter. He walked over to his truck to use his phone. Marianne lay there in the freezing cold another ten minutes until two more firemen showed up and got her into the ambulance.

The break was a bad one. She was suffering from hypothermia, and in shock. An infection set in after the operation to put pins in her badly shattered ankle. She was in bed for six months. The pain lessened but never stopped entirely. The doctors said she might never walk again without a walker. She pleaded to go to physical therapy.

"What do you think physical therapy is going to do for *you?* Look at you, what do you expect?" one of the HMO doctors said.

But Marianne insisted. And a nutritionist at the hospital befriended her. "Look," the woman said. "Don't try to diet. Eat normally, but cut all the fat out of everything you eat. I promise you, even though you're lying in bed, you'll lose."

As Marianne lay in bed day after day, worried about her job, thinking about her life, falling into despair, she began to pray to Saint Anne, her patron saint. She asked for guidance. She asked to be able to walk again, even just to be able to walk her dog. After three and a half months in bed, simply by carefully cutting the fat out of her diet, she had lost thirty pounds. She began to think there was hope.

When she went back to the hospital, demanding to be allowed to go to physical therapy, they insisted on weighing her—with a special scale, one that would register her full poundage.

Talking loudly, inconsiderate of her feelings, the orderlies remarked that they couldn't put her on the one for most of their patients. They joked with each other as if she didn't even exist.

"Remember that lady who weighed in at 325? Boy, was she big! Broke the springs."

"Oh, yeah, do I ever. We're not going through that again. No way. Took us three weeks to get another scale in here."

"Yeah. We had to walk all the way down to chemo every time we needed a goddamn scale. Hell, I finally brought in the one from my bathroom."

Marianne kept her feelings inside. She was determined to get what she had come there for. For the first time in her life, she got on a treadmill. She did everything the physical therapist asked of her. She worked hard. Soon she got rid of the walker and walked with a cane. But the pain didn't stop—and the money allotted by the insurance company for her therapy ran out.

Again she was up against a brick wall. Now, besides praying, she made a vigil to Saint Anne at the basilica in Scranton, Pennsylvania. She asked if she should just accept her disability and learn to live with it. She prayed for guidance. The answer she received was loud and clear: *Don't give up. Fight to walk again. Fight to stop the pain. Go after your dreams.* The next day, Marianne's physical therapist suggested she try to find a personal trainer and work out at the local gym.

"Oh, like Oprah Winfrey," she said, wondering how she could possibly afford it.

"Yeah," her therapist said, and added, "Look, resistance training might help you. At the very least, if you took some of the weight off the ankle, it would heal better."

As if she didn't know she had to lose pounds—as if she hadn't tried. She started calling the list of trainers she had obtained from the hospital. One by one, she ticked them off her list as she held the same phone interview over and over:

"I need someone to work with me. I had a fractured ankle. Surgery has left me with considerable pain and difficulty walking. And I have a weight problem."

"Oh yeah, how much do you weigh?"

"A significant amount."

"Well, um, I don't think I can help you. Why don't you lose some weight first, then call me back."

Discouraged, loathing herself, filled with self-hatred, and falling into despair, she forced herself to pick up the phone and call the last person on her list. At least she would know that she had tried. A man with a kind voice answered. His name was Paul, and he worked at a combination rehabilitation center and gym on the outskirts of Wilkes Barre. He asked how he could help her.

She explained about her ankle injury.

He asked her to tell him more about what she hoped to get out of working with him. Marianne took a deep breath and found she was telling him things she had never said to the others. She said she had three goals: first, to relieve her pain. Second, to walk without a cane. The third was a private dream she wasn't ready to talk about. And, oh yes: "I have a weight problem."

"Why don't you come out and see me? I think I can help you."

He never asked how much she weighed. He was the only one.

"I hobbled in with a cane. My heart was beating like a hummingbird's wings. I was so scared. I felt as if this was my last chance. Then I saw Paul standing there. He had striking, black-Irish good looks, a smile filled with sunshine, and a twinkle in his brown eyes. He was tall and muscular. *Oh no,* I thought. *This isn't going to work. Someone like that isn't going to want to work with someone like me.* I was so used to being rejected, I figured, *Why go through it again?*"

Passing by a stationary bike, stopping by a Nautilus machine, Marianne came no closer than five feet from Paul. He smiled at her, but before he could say anything, she blurted out, "I'm sorry to have wasted your time"—her voice wobbled, she thought she was going to cry—"but I can't do this. It's just not going to work." She turned around and hobbled toward the door.

Paul ran after her. "Wait, don't go! Give me a chance. I can help you. Let me at least try." He got in front of her. Marianne had to stop. He looked at her face, into her eyes. He didn't stare at her body.

"Please. Let's at least try working together," he said quietly, gently. "I won't let you get hurt. I promise not to ask you to do anything you don't feel ready for. But I'm sure I can help you."

Marianne suddenly realized that what she had just done to this nice young man with the gentle voice and kind eyes was exactly what people had done to her all her life. She had judged him on his appearance.

They began to work together. It was a collaboration that would begin the total transformation of Marianne's life.

"Food is not your enemy, Marianne," Paul said. "Food gives you energy. You have to eat, every three hours. Yes, every three hours. You don't want to get hungry. What you eat is important, too, but you *must* eat. You need to change the way you think about food."

Marianne changed. She began weight training. She did a lot of leg work to help her ankle. She began to lose weight. The pounds fell off of her—twenty pounds a month. The pain stopped. She walked without a cane

Weight training, and Paul's guidance, also put Marianne in touch with her body. Before working with Paul, Marianne had always thought of her being, her true self, as someone inside her mind, and her body as just a shell, not really part of her; it was separate from her real self. She didn't identify with it at all. She rejected it. Hell, she *hated* it. Now, Paul told her she had terrific bones. They were strong and well-shaped. He showed her how to concentrate on her muscles, to isolate the one she was working, to really feel it. One day, working on the leg-lift machine, she looked down at her thigh, and she could see the quadriceps muscle—for the first time, she could see the outline of one of her own muscles and watch it move.

Paul said, "You know, Marianne, you need to like your body. It's you. In fact, you need to love your body, because it means you can love yourself." Smart, quick, and ready to hear what Paul was saying, Marianne worked on herself emotionally and spiritually as

well as physically. And she began to love the way she could walk
and move. She felt as if she had been released from prison. She felt
light. She felt strong. She glided, she strode, she could even run.
Soon, loving herself, too, didn't seem so impossible.

In less than a year, going to the gym five times a week, Marianne dropped from 320 pounds to 165 pounds. She now weighs
145, and wears a size 6. She didn't starve herself. She ate "clean," as
the weight lifters say. She chose whole, fresh foods, kept her fat
intake very low, chose complex carbohydrates, and cut out all
junk foods. She never skipped a meal or snack; she made sure she
ate regularly. Her metabolism speeded up. As the inches disappeared, Paul never asked how much she was losing. He never
asked how much she weighed. And then he told her he was relo-
cating to the Midwest. She felt as if he was cutting her heart out.
She feared that without him, she couldn't do it. What if she started
gaining weight again?

"Marianne," Paul said in his quiet way, "I need to go, and I need
to let you go, so you can grow. We've come this far together, but you
are strong enough to make the rest of the journey without me."

She was ready to go on. And before Paul left, they had a frank
talk about one thing no one had ever told her about weight loss: Its
effect on her skin. "You know, Marianne," Paul explained, "your
skin isn't going to retract. The job of fat is to support the skin.
When you remove the support, the skin falls—and you have all the
skin that you started with a year ago. The body doesn't reabsorb it.
The only way to get rid of it is surgery. Or you can live with it."

Marianne couldn't live with it. Paul didn't know how horrific
the problem had become. The skin on Marianne's legs drooped in
multiple folds down past her knees. She had to wear tights or
pantyhose to keep it from sliding down her legs. Marianne's arms
had always been big—even bigger than her thighs. Now they were
hideous-looking. She had to wear long, tight sleeves to contain over
a foot of loose skin that hung beneath each arm. Her body looked

as if she had melted, the flesh rolled downward in drooping folds. She became a master of disguise, carefully choosing clothes to cover the bumps and rolls. She tried to avoid anyone touching her, for fear they would discover the yards of skin she had tucked into Spandex and Lycra. A friendly hug? Not for the "ice maiden," as people at work began to call her. She'd pull back even if someone tried to put an arm around her shoulder. She was untouchable. No one knew how much she ached to be touched, to be held, to feel the comfort of strong arms around her.

But the truth was, she looked like a freak without her clothes. She needed surgery if she was going to have any hope of a normal life. But her insurance company said no. She had asked, she had pleaded, she had even been sent to a two-hour "tribunal" in front of a panel of doctors at a major medical center hours from her home.

It was like the Spanish Inquisition. Marianne sat in a chair facing a long table. Behind the table sat her judges, dressed in white and carrying clipboards or manila folders. Many of the questioners were women. None of them smiled. They asked if she could walk. "Yes." Was she still in pain? "No." They commented that she looked normal, even attractive. She carefully explained her problem. She showed them the skin on her arms. She lifted her skirt, feeling totally humiliated, to show the drapes of skin on her legs. They were medical people, and they knew the health risks of having such large amounts of excess skin, including ulceration and infection. Yet the bottom line ruled—and so did something else that Marianne still didn't know about. Very few surgeons did this sort of surgery. Protocols didn't even exist for many of the procedures she would need. Her surgery would be, in a very real way, "experimental." The stony-faced answer from Marianne's judges that day was, "No."

"You can walk," they said. "You can live a normal life with your clothes on."

But Marianne wanted more than a life "with her clothes on." She wanted to put on pair of shorts in the summer, even a bathing suit. She wanted to hike and swim. But more than that. She wanted her dreams: the boyfriend, the lover, the chance for marriage and babies. Men were asking her out, but she said no. She did look attractive—with her clothes on. But her appearance without clothes was what she called "the elephant woman." She felt that becoming involved with a man at this point would be dishonest. She would be misleading someone. And the thought of rejection by someone she cared about when he saw her without clothes was unbearable. No one had ever seen her without clothes. It was her secret.

Turning again to prayer, fighting the darkness with the guiding light of Saint Anne, Marianne asked to be shown a way to health and wholeness. "Some surgeons will perform operations pro bono," a doctor mentioned to her one day. "It can't hurt to ask."

Swallowing one's pride does hurt. Begging does hurt. Rejection does hurt. But feeling strong enough to bear that pain to get what she needed, Marianne began asking well-known surgeons for help. One by one—sometimes kindly, sometimes not—surgeons shut their doors to her. The answer was always a firm no.

I don't know what made me call the Renaissance Center. Except that the name called to me. It reflected my own quest for rebirth and renewal. And I don't know what made me ask who handled the business end of the practice.

"Dr. Collini's wife," the receptionist said. I asked if I could come in to see her—and, wonder of wonders, they checked with her, and she said to come in.

When I first saw Susan, I was even more frightened than I had been when I made the phone call. I saw this physically perfect, beautiful, truly radiant woman sitting behind a desk. She looked like someone in the movies, only here she was, real, in front of me. But her voice was all kindness. I was so afraid to tell her about my problem, so afraid to hear her say no.

I took a deep breath, and my story just rushed out. I told her how no doctor would help me; in fact no one could help me. Susan listened to me intently. She never interrupted. When I stopped talking, she got up from her chair and came around the desk. She put her arms around me and held me. Then she said, "We will not abandon you. We will help you."

Marianne didn't know that Dr. Collini was one of the few surgeons who was not only willing to do this difficult surgery, but had had considerable experience in doing it successfully. She couldn't have known of his extensive pro bono work in the jungle cities of Ecuador each year. She couldn't have known that both Susan and Dr. Collini are committed Roman Catholics. Marianne couldn't have known, but perhaps Saint Anne did.

Marianne and Susan worked out a plan for payment, one that is known only between them. The cost of the surgeries was over $100,000. Yes, it cost more than most individuals can afford in a lifetime. Yes, these are surgeries that insurance companies should pay for, that women should begin to lobby for and insist that HMOs pay for.

But money was only one obstacle Marianne had to cross. She didn't want to take her clothes off in front of Dr. Collini.

No one had ever seen me naked. I pleaded with the doctor to just knock me out and look at me when I was on the table. I didn't want to see what his reaction would be. I didn't want to see his face when he saw me. But he was so kind. He explained that he needed to examine me or he couldn't help me. He was so careful to preserve my modesty when he did look, draping my body and keeping any eyes but his from seeing me. He was very sensitive to my feelings, and just so very kind. I guess "I have always depended on the kindness of strangers," but I don't want to be like Blanche DuBois, she added, about this famous line from *A Streetcar Named Desire.* That character's inner pain strikes too close to my heart than is healthy.

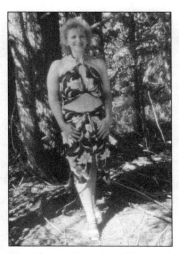

Magnificent and courageous Marianne Korey dares to bare her new bellybutton after skin reduction surgeries on her arms, tummy, thighs, and sides! May all her dreams come true.

Marianne also found the tremendous courage to undergo the extensive reconstructive procedures she needed to reduce her skin. (Anyone who would like to read in detail about the surgeries, can look up Dr. Collini's article, published in *Perspectives in Plastic Surgery*, and reference "case 11.") A series of sequential surgeries over the course of a year reshaped her thighs, her buttocks, her back, her stomach, her breasts, her arms. She even had her nose reshaped to fit her new, smaller face. Sometimes she was on the operating table for over five hours. The skin on her arms was so extensive, she had to have them operated on twice. Yards of skin were removed, all while she was under safe intravenous sedation and local anesthesia, *not* general anesthesia.

She emerged after months of surgery with an hourglass figure— a knockout.

"I didn't know what I was supposed to look like," she said. "I had never seen a naked woman, and I had never looked normal. I didn't know what a man looked like, either! I truly didn't know— embarrassing as that seems. I went out and bought a *Playboy* magazine and a *Playgirl* magazine to see what normal bodies looked like. I really did."

"Marianne," Dr. Collini smiled, as he lectured her. "You don't need to look at those magazines. You don't have to look like those girls. You have to find your own beauty."

"And I have. You know what I love best?" she said. "My belly button. You have to understand, I never had a belly button before. When I was heavy, it was lost in the fat. When I lost weight it was just a huge crease between the folds of skin. Now I feel normal—and look wonderful. How wonderful? I wear crop tops and show it off as much as I can. Dr. Collini is a Michelangelo, I mean that. The belly button he created is beautiful. Once I had a crop top on under my shirt at work. Unknown to me, the buttons had opened. I was zooming around the office with my usual energy, when finally one of the young guys at work came up and whined, 'Mer…'

"'What's the matter, Ronnie?' I asked.

"'Mer, you have to button your shirt. You're driving us crazy over here. We can't concentrate. All we can do is stare at you, and we're not getting any work done. We're just guys, you know. We can't help it!'"

Marianne could hardly believe her ears.

A few weeks later, this happened:

"Mer . . ."

"Yes, Ronnie?"

"The guys held an informal vote in the office for the prettiest woman and the best-built woman. You won."

"Won what?" Marianne asked, flabbergasted.

"Both, Mer. You won both!"

"Fatty, fatty."

Sometimes Marianne is still haunted by those memories, but no longer does the world see a woman hidden in a mountain of fat. Thanks to her own determination, and the skills of a great surgeon, they see someone as beautiful on the outside as she is inside, a woman with hopes that can now be fulfilled, who wrote this.

My Essence as a Woman
by Marianne Korey

(dedicated to Susan and Francis Collini who have helped to silence the voices)

They did not see the beauty within me, the treasures of my soul.
I searched for the healing powers to quiet their voices.

And rediscover the jewels that lay broken and buried.
Trusting the sculptor's hands I reveled in his magic
To reshape the shrine of a hungry heart reaching out for help.
The voices of a painful past grow faint, as I become fit and strong.
I pay no heed to the voices of the present that try to darken my journey.

I hug myself as I look intently in the mirror,
Silencing the wild dogs in my mind,
Soothing the battle wounds that I can see and the scars deep within me.
This is a face with glistening blue eyes
That embraces life with childlike wonder.
This is a body illuminating with warmth
From full breasts and shapely hips.
Mine is the scent of softness carried on a gentle breeze.
Mine is the laughter that bubbles from within an open, giving heart.
Each day I am new, reborn, and more at peace with myself.
I reclaim, moment by moment, my own special treasures,
No longer empowering the voices to define me, mold me, hurt me.
I forgive them, I forgive myself, learning when to let go.
It is I, not the voices, who will create my world.

The beauty of my soul has transcended time,
Surviving the pain of a physical image ridiculed by many.
I unearthed and polished my jewels, healing my mind, body, and spirit,
Rescuing my beauty, becoming the woman I was always meant to be.
The voices become still as I raise graceful arms above my head.
Dancing barefoot in the moon's silver rays,
I move to the sweet melody within me.
Gazing up at the blue-white crystals in the midnight sky
I dream of a lover who will discover
My essence as a woman that is warm and rich with treasures.

BIBLIOGRAPHY

Achauer, Bruce M. "ASAPS/ASPRS Laser Task Force Report." *Aesthetic Surgery Quarterly*. Spring 1996, 32–34.

Adamson, Peter A. "Rhinoplasty—Our Past." *Facial Plastic Surgery*. Winter 1988, vol. 5, no. 2, 93–96.

Anastasi, Gaspar W., et al. "Minimal Breast Reduction and Mastoplexy." *Aesthetic Surgery Journal*. Fall 1995, 4–10.

Anderson, Rebecca Cogwell. "Aesthetic Surgery and Pyschosexual Issues." *Aesthetic Surgery Quarterly*. Winter 1996, 227–28.

Apfelberg, David B. "UltraPulse Carbon Dioxide Laser with CPB Scanner for Full-Face Resurfacing for Rhytids, Photoaging, and Acne Scars." *Plastic and Reconstructive Surgery*. June 1997, vol. 99, no. 7, 1819, 1822–23.

Baack, Bret R., et al. "Umbilicoplasty: The Construction of a New Umbilicus and Correction of Umbilical Stenosis without External Scars." *Plastic and Reconstructive Surgery*. January 1996, vol. 97, no. 1, 231.

Baker, Thomas J., and Stuzin, James M. "Personal Technique of Face-lifting." *Plastic and Reconstructive Surgery*. August 1997, vol. 100, no. 2, 504–8.

Baroudi, R. "Umbilicoplasty." *Clinical Plastic Surgery*. 1975, 2:431.

Barton, Fritz E., and Gyimesi, Ildiko M. "Anatomy of the Nasolabial Fold." *Plastic and Reconstructive Surgery.* October 1997, 1276–80.

Bates, H. K., et al. "Developmental Toxicity Evaluation of the Mammary Implant, Silicone Gel P/N 3200, Implanted Subcutaneously in Rats." *Toxicologist.* 1993, 13:381.

Beninger, Francis Gregory, and Pritchard, Sandy James. "Clonidine in the Management of Blood Pressure During Rhytidectomy." *Aesthetic Surgery Journal.* March/April 1998, volume 18, no. 2, 89–94.

Benvenuti, David. "Necrosis of the Nasal Tip." *Plastic and Reconstructive Surgery.* July 1995, vol. 96, no. 1, 223–4.

Berkel, H., et al. "Breast Augmentation: A Risk Factor for Breast Cancer?" *New England Journal of Medicine.* 1992, 326:1649–53.

Brody G. S., et al. "Consensus Statement on the Relationship of Breast Implants to Connective-Tissue Disorders." *Plastic and Reconstructive Surgery.* 1992, 90:1102–05.

Byrd, H. Steve. "The Dimensional Approach to Rhinoplasty: Perfecting the Aesthetic Balance Between the Nose and Chin." Rhinoplasty Symposium, 1994, 33–39.

Byrd, H. Steve, and Andochick, Scott E. "The Deep Temporal Lift: A Multiplanar, Lateral Brow, Temporal, and Upper Face-lift." *Plastic and Reconstructive Surgery.* April 1996, vol. 97, no. 5, 928–37.

Caputy, Gregory. "The Computer and Truth." *Plastic and Reconstructive Surgery.* February 1994, vol. 93, no. 2, 393–95.

Cohen, Marsha M. "Does Anesthesia Contribute to Operative Mortality?" *JAMA.* November 18, 1988, vol. 260, no. 19, 2859.

Collini, Francis J. "Profiles in Skin Reduction Surgery." *Perspectives in Plastic Surgery.* 1999, vol. 13, 83–135.

Colton, Jeffrey J., and Beekhuis, G. Jan. "Presurgical Analysis for Rhinoplasty." *Facial Plastic Surgery.* Winter 1988, vol. 5, no. 2, 97–107.

Connell, Bruce F. and Shamoun, John M. "The Significance of Digastric Muscle Contouring for Rejuvenation of the Submental Area of the Face." *Plastic and Reconstructive Surgery.* May 1997, vol. 99, no. 6, 1586–90.

"Cosmetic Surgery: The Hidden Dangers." *Sun-Sentinel.* December 2, 198, 27A.

Deapen, D. M., and Brody, G. S. "Augmentation Mammaplasty and Breast Cancer: A 5-Year Update of the Los Angeles Study." *Plastic and Reconstructive Surgery.* 1992, 89:660–65.

————. The Los Angeles breast implant cancer study update: 15–20 year follow-up. Presented to the ASPRS Annual Meeting; September 21, 1993, New Orleans, LA.

Deapen, D. M., et al. "The Relationship between Breast Cancer and Augmentation Mammaplasty: An Epidemiologic Study." *Plastic and Reconstructive Surgery.* 1986, 77:361–68.

"Disease—Clinical and Immunological Investigations." *Arthritis and Rheumatology.* 1992, 35:S65, Abstract.

Duffy, David M., M.D. "Alpha-Hydroxy Acids/Tricholoroacetic Acids: Risk/Benefit Strategies." *American Society for Dermatologic Surgery, Inc.* 1998, 181.

Editorial, *Aesthetic Surgery Journal.* September/October 1997, 316.

Elson, Melvin L. "Topical Phytonadione (Vitamin K1) in the Treatment of Actinic and Traumatic Purpura." *Cosmetic Dermatology.* December 1995, vol. 8, no. 12, 25–27.

Engel, A., et al. "Risks of Sarcomas of the Breast among Women with Breast Augmentation." *Plastic and Reconstructive Surgery.* 1992, 89:571–572.

Epstein, Emily, et al. "Prospective and Randomized Determination of the Efficacy of Topical Lipolytic Agents." *Aesthetic Surgery Journal.* September/October 1997, 304–7.

Ersek, Robert A., and Burry, Heidi. "Persistent Pigmentation: A Complication of Liposuction." *Aesthetic Plastic Surgery.* 1995, 19:379-80.

Ersek, Robert A., and Salisbury, A.V. "Circumferential Liposuction of Knees, Calves, and Ankles." *Plastic and Reconstructive Surgery.* October 1996, 880–83.

FDA information for women considering saline-filled breast implants. *McGhan Medical Corporation.* 1995: 2.

Feeney, Sheila Anne, and Ferraro, Susan. "Make Sure Your Surgeon's a Cut Above." *New York Daily News.* August 18, 1998.

Fodor, Peter Bela, and Watson, James. "Personal Experience with Ultrasound-Assisted Lipoplasty: A Pilot Study Comparing Ultrasound-Assisted Lipoplasty with Traditional Lipoplasty." *Plastic and Reconstructive Surgery.* April 1998, 1103–19.

Gabriel, S. E., et al. "Risk of Connective-Tissue Diseases and Other Disorders After Breast Implantation." *New England Journal of Medicine.* 1994, 330:1697–1702.

Garner, D. M. "The 1997 Body Image Survey Results." *Psychology Today.* 1997, 31:30–84.

Glass, Leonard W. "Subperiosteal Face-Lift: A Mid Face Degloving Technique Through an Intraoral Approach." *Aesthetic Surgery Journal.* March/April 1997, 124–32.

Goddio, A. S. "Skin Retraction Following Suction Lipectomy by Treatment Site: A Study of 500 Procedures in 458 Selected Subjects." *Plastic and Reconstructive Surgery.* January 1991, 66–75.

Goin, M. K., et al. "A Prospective Psychological Study of 50 Female Face-Lift Patients." *Plastic and Reconstructive Surgery.* 1980, vol. 65, 436–42.

Grazer, Frederick M. "Late Bleeding from the Superficial Temporal Vessels after Rhytidectomy." *Plastic and Reconstructive Surgery.* April 1992, vol. 89, no. 4, 767.

Gruber, Ronald P., and Jones, Hyzer W., Jr. "The 'Donut' Mastoplexy: Indications and Complications." *Plastic and Reconstructive Surgery.* January 1980, vol. 65, no. 1, 34–38.

Guyuron, Bahman, and Zarandy, Simin. "Does Rhinoplasty Make the Nose More Suspectible to Fracture?" *Plastic and Reconstructive Surgery.* February 1994, vol. 93, no. 2, 313–17.

Guyuron, Bahman, et al. "Secondary Rhytidectomy." *Plastic and Reconstructive Surgery.* October 1997, vol. 100, no. 5, 1281–83.

Hage, J. Joris, et al. "Gender-Confirming Facial Surgery: Considerations on the Masculinity and Femininity of Faces." *Plastic and Reconstructive Surgery.* June 1997, vol. 99, no. 7, 1799–1806.

Hamilton, John M. "Submental Lipectomy with Skin Excision." *Plastic and Reconstructive Surgery.* September 1994, vol. 92, no. 3, 443–48.

Hamilton, John M. and Bowell, Michelle. "My Experience with 3,500 Face-lifts." *Aesthetic Surgery Quarterly.* Fall 1996, 205–7.

Hamra, Sam T. "Surgery of the Aging Chin." *Plastic and Reconstructive Surgery.* August 1994, vol. 94, no. 2, 388–93.

Har-Shai, Yaron, et al. "Mechanical Properties and Microstructure of the Superficial Musculoaponeurotic System." *Plastic and Reconstructive Surgery.* July 1996, vol. 98, no. 1, 59–70.

Hester, T. Roderick, Jr., et al. "Abdominoplasty Combined with Other Major Surgical Procedures: Safe or Sorry?" *Plastic and Reconstructive Surgery.* June 1989, vol. 83, no. 6, 997–1003.

Hochberg, M. C., et al. "The Association of Augmentation Mammaplasty With Systemic Sclerosis: Results From a Multi-Center Case-Control Study." *Arthritis and Rheumatology.* 1994, 37:S369, Abstract.

Hoefflin, Steven M. "Facial Rejuvenation—My Personal Evolution." *Aesthetic Surgery Journal.* July/August 1998, 286–89.

Horton, Charles E. "Aesthetic Rhinoplasty: My Perspectives." *Aesthetic Surgery Journal.* May/June 1997, 170–74.

Hurwitz, Dennis, and Raskin, Elsa M. "Reducing Eyelid Retraction Following Subperiosteal Face-lift." *Aesthetic Surgery Journal.* May/June 1997, 149–56.

Jan Marini Skin Research Resource Manual, "Photodamage/Aging Skin," 4.

Joas, Thomas A. "Sedation and Anesthesia in the Office Setting." *Aesthetic Surgery Journal.* July/August 1998, 300–301.

Jones, Barry M. "The Late Bleeding Face-lift (Re)Visited." *Plastic and Reconstructive Surgery.* August 1998, 577.

Kaye, Bernard L. "Discussion: Restoration of the Upper Lip and Nasolabial Area by Means of an Intraoral Approach." *Plastic and Reconstructive Surgery.* October 1986, vol. 78, no. 4, 457–59.

Kaye, Bernard L. "The Pre-sideburn Incision Preserves the Sideburn." *Aesthetic Surgery Journal.* May/June 1997, 196, 198.

Kaye, Bernard L., et al. "Panel Discussion: Complications of Face-lift Surgery." *Aesthetic Surgery Journal.* January/February 1998.

Kennedy, G. L., et al. "Reproductive, Teratologuc, and Mutagenic Studies with Some Polydimethylsiloxanes." *Journal of Toxicology and Environmental Health.* 1976, 1:909–20.

Kolar, Amy. "The Role of the Nurse in Intravenous Dissociative Anesthesia." *Plastic Surgery Nursing.* Summer 1983, 29–31.

Kotzur, Annette, and Gubisch, Wolfgang. "Mucous Cyst—A Postrhinoplasty Complication: Outcome and Prevention." *Plastic and Reconstructive Surgery.* August 1997, vol. 100, no. 2, 520–24.

Krastinova-Lolov, Darina. "Mask Lift and Facial Aesthetic Sculpturing." *Plastic and Reconstructive Surgery.* January 1995, vol. 95, no. 1, 21–36.

Lai, Y. L., et al. "Areolar Reduction with Inner Doughnut Incision." *Plastic and Reconstructive Surgery.* May 1998, vol. 101, no. 6, 1695–99.

LeRoy, Laura. "Laser Resurfacing: The Nurse's Role." *Dermatology Nursing.* June 1997, vol. 9, no. 3, 173.

Lesavoy, Malcolm, et al. "A Technique for Correcting Witch's Chin Deformity." *Plastic and Reconstructive Surgery.* April 1996, vol. 97, no. 4, 449–46.

Lillis, Patrick J. "Liposuction: How Aggressive Should It Be?" *Tumescent Liposuction Council Bulletin.* 1996, 973–76.

Maillard, G. F., et al. "The Subperiosteal Bicoronal Approach to Total Face-lifting: The DMAS—Deep Musculoaponeurotic System." *Aesthetic Plastic Surgery.* 1991, 15:285–91.

Marconi, Franco, and Cavina, Carlo. "Reduction Mammaplasty and Correction of Ptosis: A Personal Technique." *Plastic and Reconstructive Surgery.* May 1993, vol. 191, no. 6, 1046–56.

Matory, W. Earle, et al. "Abdominal Surgery in Patients with Severe Morbid Obesity." *Plastic and Reconstructive Surgery.* December 1994, vol. 94, no. 7, 976–87.

May, James W., Jr. "Preoperative and Postoperative Care for Patients Undergoing Blepharoplasty and Face-lift." *Aesthetic Surgery Journal.* May/June 1997, 192–94.

Mayl, Nathan, M.D. "Management of Facial Telangiectasia and Vascular Visibility." *Aesthetic Surgery Quarterly.* Fall 1996, vol. 16, no. 3, 164, 166.

Menz, Peter. "Pregnancy after Abdominoplasty." *Plastic and Reconstructive Surgery.* August 1996, vol. 98, no. 2, 377–78.

Millard, Ralph, et al. "A Challenge to the Undefeated Nasolabial Folds." *Plastic and Reconstructive Surgery.* July 1987, vol. 80, no. 1, 37–46.

Miller, Timothy A., and Orringer, Jay S. "Excision of Neck Redundancy with Single Z-Plasty Closure." *Plastic and Reconstructive Surgery.* January 1996, vol. 97, no. 1, 219–21.

Moscona, Rony A., et al. "A Comparison of Sedation Techniques for Outpatient Rhinoplasty: Midazolam versus Midazolam plus Ketamine." *Plastic and Reconstructive Surgery.* October 1995, vol. 96, no. 5, 1066–74.

Muhanna, A., et al. "Silicone Breast Implants and Rheumatic Disease—Clinical and Immunological Investigations." *Arthritis and Rheumatology.* 1992, 35:S65, Abstract

Mühlbauer, Wolfgang. "Radical Abdominoplasty, Including Body Shaping: Representative Cases." *Aesthetic Plastic Surgery.* 1989, 13:105–10.

O'Donoghue, Marianne N. "New Camouflaging Technique following Laser Resurfacing." *Dermatological Surgery (CK).* 1997, 23:717–18.

Owsley, John. Q. "Face-lift." *Plastic and Reconstructive Surgery.* August 1997, vol. 100, no. 2, 514–19.

Paloma, Vicente, et al. "A Simple Device for Marking the Areola in Lejour's Mammaplasty." *Plastic and Reconstructive Surgery.* November 1998, vol. 102, no. 6, 2134–38.

Panel discussion by Rod Rohrich, et al. *Aesthetic Surgery Quarterly.* Winter 1996, 218–23.

Panel discussion, "Treatment of Postlaser Resurfacing Complications." *Aesthetic Surgery Journal.* March/April 1997, 122.

Panel discussion. "Ultrasound-Assisted Lipoplasty and Suction-Assisted Lipoplasty." *Aesthetic Surgery Journal.* May/June 1997, 181–87.

Pensler, Jay M., et al. "Restoration of the Upper Lip and Nasolabial Area by Means of an Intraoral Approach." *Plastic and Reconstructive Surgery.* October 1986, vol. 78, no. 4, 449–56.

Preston, Lydia. "Laser Surgery Before 40." *Self.* July 1997, 129–34.

Ramirez, Oscar M. and Pozner, Jason N. "Subperiosteal Endoscopic Techniques in Secondary Rhytidectomy." *Aesthetic Surgery Journal.* January/February 1997, 22–28.

Rees, Thomas D., et al. "Hematomas Requiring Surgical Evacuation Following Face-lift Surgery." *Plastic and Reconstructive Surgery.* May 1994, vol. 93, no. 6, 1185–90.

Rohrich, Rod J., and DiSpaltra, Franklin L. "Potential Long-Term Effects of Ultrasound-Assisted Lipoplasty: A Clinical Analysis." *Aesthetic Surgery Journal.* July/August 1998, 271–73.

Rosenbaum, Michael, et al. "An Exploratory Investigation of the Morphology and Biochemistry of Cellulite." *Plastic and Reconstructive Surgery.* June 1998, 1934–39.

Sanchez-Guerrero, J., et al. "Silicone Breast Implants and Connective Tissue Disease." *Arthritis and Rheumatology.* 1994, 37:S282, Abstract.

———. "Silicone Breast Implants and Rheumatic Disease. Clinical, Immunologic, and Epidemiologic Studies." *Arthritis and Rheumatology.* 1994, 37:158–168.

Sarwer, David B., et al. "Body Image Dissatisfaction in Women Seeking Rhytidectomy or Blepharoplasty." *Aesthetic Surgery Journal.* July/August 1997, 230–34.

Sarwar, David B., et al. "Psychological Investigations in Cosmetic Surgery: A Look Back and a Look Ahead." *Plastic and Reconstructive Surgery.* April 1998, vol. 101, no. 4, 1136–40.

Schulte, Fred, and Bergal, Jenni. "Marketing Blitz Entices Patients." *Fort Lauderdale Sun-Sentinel.* December 1, 1998; 1, 10A.

Seckel, Flossie R. "Aesthetic Laser Surgery," *Dow Hickam Pharmaceuticals, Inc.* Little, Brown, and Company, 1996.

Self. July, 1997, p. 131

Sheen, Jack H. "Rhinoplasty and Mentoplasty." *Patient Care in Specific Types of Plastic Surgery,* vol. II, chapter 13, 153–61.

Slavin, Sumner A., et al. "Minimal Incision Breast Surgery." *Aesthetic Surgery Journal.* September/October 1998, 361–69.

Spiera, R. F., et al. "Silcone Gel Filled Breast Implants and Connective Tissue Disease: An Overview." *Journal of Rheumatology.* 1994, 21:239–45.

Terino, Edward. "Identifying the Dangerous Patient." American Society for Plastic and Reconstructive Surgeons Symposium, 1993.

Topaz, Morris. "Possible Long-Term Complications in Ultrasound-Assisted Lipoplasty, Induced Sonoluminescence, Sonochemistry, and Thermal Effect." *Aesthetic Surgery Journal.* January/February 1998, 19–24.

Toranto, I. Richard. "The Relief of Low Back Pain with the WARP Abdominoplasty: A Preliminary Report." *Plastic and Reconstructive Surgery.* vol. 85, no. 4, 545–55.

Weinstein, Cynthia, et al. "Complications of Carbon Dioxide Laser Resurfacing and Their Prevention." *Aesthetic Surgery Journal.* July/August 1997, 216–25.

Yoshida, S. H., et al. "Silicon and Silicone: Theoretical and Clinical Implications of Breast Implants." *Regulations of Toxicology and Pharmacology.* 1993, 17:3–18.

INDEX

Index   311

sinus problems, 179, 268

ski nose, 180

skin cancer, 185, 186

skin necrosis, 137

skin reduction, 61–62, 68–72, 104, 106, 116, 271–291

skin, 68–69, 79, 131, 145, 169, 179, 185–201, 203–208, 209–220

sleep disorders, 41

sleep tips for recovery, 192, 257–258

smoking, 120, 137, 164, 185, 246, 258

sneezing and rhinoplasty, 176

splints and tape after rhinoplasty, 175, 177

statistics regarding plastic surgery, xx, 45, 94, 127, 187, 203, 215, 217, 218

stenosis, 74

steroid drugs and products, 137, 143, 178, 251

stitch abscesses, 144

stretch marks, 208

strong chins, 168

subdermal therapy, 65–66

suction-assisted lipoplasty, 48

sun damage, 58, 140, 155, 177, 185, 186, 191, 193, 194, 197, 204, 206, 208, 215

superficial temporal artery, 144

surgeons, 62, 80, 172–174, 187–188, 207, 225, 226–227, 229, 230–236

surgery, xi, xiii, xxiii, 31–42, 45–66, 52–57, 103–104, 116, 136–139, 151–159, 203–204, 232, 245–250, 247–248, 250–259, 269–291

surgical facilities, 227–228, 235, 236

sutures after surgery, 120, 152, 154, 155, 164

swelling after surgery, 59, 104, 105, 118, 142, 155, 157, 160, 164, 165, 167, 168, 172, 178, 179, 190, 204, 205, 210, 220, 251, 257

-T-

tear duct injury, 179–180

tearing or dry eyes, 157

telangiectasia, 179, 186, 192, 215

temporary parotid fistula, 144

temporary wrinkle removal, 218

thighplasty, 46–47, 50, 88

thighs, xvii, 46, 50, 51

tightness, 142, 164

"tits on a stick," 94

transfusions, 48, 55, 119–120

tretonin, *see* Retin-A

trichloroacetic acid (TCA) peels, 210, 211, 215

trade-offs, 53–54, 60–63, 80–81, 85, 88, 89–90, 121, 147, 161, 165, 186–187, 214–215,

Trump, Ivana, 161

tumescent technique, 54

tummies, xvii, 67–81

tummy tuck,

belly button reconstruction and, 74

combined with other abdominal surgery, 73

complications, 79–80, 246

conditions fixed by, 68–72, 74

cover story for, 263, 266

exercise and, 76, 79

figure of incision, 73

"the garment" and, 75

girlfriends' tips for recovering safely from, 75

making the decision, 81

obesity and, 69, 80

personal story of, 46–47

pregnancy after, 80

recovery time for, 75–79

scars and, 80

surgical procedures of, 73–75

when to call your doctor, 75, 78

turkey wattles, 128, 192

twilight sleep, 254

-U-

ulnar nerve compression and oversized breasts, 116

ultrasound-assisted lipoplasty (UAL), 48, 53, 51–52

About the Authors

CHARLEE IRENE GANNY has been the principal in Writers Unlimited, Inc., a copywriting and editorial services business for New York and West Coast publishers, since 1984. Originally from the New York metropolitan area and now living in northeast Pennsylvania, Charlee has a bachelor's degree Magna Cum Laude with Honors in English from Drew University and a master's degree in English literature from Rutgers University. She did post-graduate study in English at Princeton University after receiving a National Endowment for the Humanities Fellowship. For more than a decade, Charlee was a tenured professor in humanities at Essex College in Newark, New Jersey. She also worked with students in a supportive role, as director of tutorial services for Misericordia College in Pennsylvania. She left her positions to pursue her writing career. In addition, she is a past member of the Adlerian Society of North America and has a broad background in psychology.

Her poetry and short stories have appeared in small-press magazines here and in Europe, and she is the author of *Beautiful Baby Names from Your Favorite TV Soap Opera* (written as Charlee Irene Trantino). She is currently working on a fiction project scheduled to be finished in the summer of 2000. And since she loves hunting for treasures at flea markets, yard sales, and auctions, in 1998 she also opened the Big Red Barn, a shop specializing in American antiques and collectibles.

Though Charlee has three dogs, ten cats, and assorted wildlife, she still manages to travel to Sicily and southern Italy as often as she can. As for cosmetic surgery, she is "high maintenance" whenever finances allow—from lifts to peels to tucks!

SUSAN J. COLLINI, RT®, RDMS, RDCS graduated from the Johns Hopkins School of Radiologic Technology and the Johns Hopkins School of Ultrasound. She later worked in both the trauma unit and as a full-time ultrasonographer at Johns Hopkins before becoming the program director of the Ultrasound School at St. Barnabas Hospital in Livingston, New Jersey. Her performance in the field was so outstanding that she worked with the Certifying Agency for Allied Health Programs, a division of the Joint Review Committee for Diagnostic Medical Sonography, to accredit other ultrasound programs across the country. Since 1994 she has been the business manager for the Renaissance Center for Plastic and Reconstructive Surgery, Dr. Francis J. Collini's thriving practice, and the owner of Age of Innocence, a full-service day spa and skin rejuvenation center. In 1998 she also opened Susan's Secrets, a clothing boutique. Susan's job at the Renaissance Center includes doing pre-op and post-op consultations with cosmetic surgery clients, dealing with fees and services, and listening compassionately to client concerns, hopes, and questions about the surgery. Her medical background, direct experience with thousands of cosmetic surgery patients, and first-hand experiences with her own surgery make her a unique and irreplaceable source of information. An active sportswoman as well, she exercises daily, rides her horse as often as possible, skis in the winter, and scuba dives in the summer. She and her husband, Francis J. Collini, have two children, Lauren and Joey.

FRANCIS J. COLLINI, M.D., F.A.C.S., born and raised in Brooklyn, New York, did his undergraduate work at Columbia University, his internship and residency in general surgery at Johns Hopkins Hospital and his residency in plastic surgery at the Mayo Clinic. After participating in group practices in Beverly Hills, California, and Wilkes Barre, Pennsylvania, Dr. Collini entered solo practice, where about 75 percent of his surgeries are cosmetic. Certified by the American Board of Surgery and the American Board of Plastic Surgery, Dr. Collini has published extensively in the field of plastic surgery, and is part of Hands Healing Hearts, a humanitarian effort by Dr. Collini and other surgeons who give part of their vacation time each year on a medical mission to the needy of Ecuador, South America.